WELCOME TO MENDOCINO
California's New Gold Coast
by Robert W. Matson

DEDICATED TO MOM and POP

PRAISE GOD This book is dedicated to all the "mom & pop" businesses who support and serve the visitors and residents of the Mendocino Coast. Also featured are a few compassionate non - profits who nurture and save lives - plant, animal and human. Indeed they feed the body and feed the SOUL.

PRICES & CHANGES: All listings in the various sections of this book were cross-checked for accuracy; however, the Publisher cannot guarantee the compilers' correctness of the information furnished them or the absence of errors. Prices mentioned in the features are subject to change due to fluctuations in the economy and management. Operating hours are also subject to change, especially on a seasonal basis in rural areas. As a rule of thumb, room rates may increase $5 - $10 per room per year.

45 YEARS of QUALITY: *Since 1975 Robert W. Matson has been publishing regional travel books of exceptional quality. Books that are extremely concentrated with valuable information and more than fairly priced. "Everything I write about I experience first hand," he states. The Mendocino Dining and Lodging Guide is his 6th title in the North of San Francisco Travel Series - bringing the total to over a 100,000 books in print!*

In order to participate in this book each destination had to pass specific criteria established by the author, Robert W. Matson. Each destination is exceptional in one way or another. Quality and profits go hand in hand; that way the consumer is assured of a top notch guide book to the best, whether moderate or expensive; accommodations, restaurants, galleries, general stores and select and productive non-profits North of San Francisco.

COVER PHOTOGRAPH: Veteran photographer John Birchard of Mendocino caught the sunrise of Big River Estero with this photo. His website and spectacular photos can be explored at http://www.birchardphoto.com. The **Inside Front Cover Photo** of the redwood forest and mushrooms is from Jon Klein. His spectacular photos can be seen at http://jonkleinphoto.com/

COVER DESIGN: by Robert W. Matson, http://www.northofsf.com/contact

North of San Francisco Guide Book ™
The Mendocino Dining and Lodging Guide
First Edition: Fall of 2021, Second Edition: Spring 2024
Third Edition: Spring 2026
Printed in California on partial recycled paper.
ISBN: 978-0-916310-00-4

TABLE OF CONTENTS

NOTE: The various destinations in this book appear in the order in which they are located along the highways; from south to north and east to west.

WELCOME To California's New Gold Coast!

CHAPTER ONE Feed the Body
Coastline: Albion to Westport

CHAPTER TWO Feed the Soul

WELCOME!
To The Mendocino Dining and Lodging Guide, Albion to Westport. California's New Gold Coast!

HOW TO USE THIS BOOK by Robert W. Matson

Over four decades of travel and contact with knowledgeable residents and curious visitors to the north coast have helped to field test and engineer this practical, unpretentious and easy-to-use guide book. This book is divided into two chapters. This is the first guidebook where I have deliberately partnered over 125 for profit "mom and pop" businesses with non profit organizations who provide a safety net for the less fortunate or in case of wildfire, earthquake or tsunami. The alphabetized index beginning on Page 74 lists destinations by page number. Individual destinations follow the highways in geological order, from south to north and/or east to west. Happy Trails!

PRICES and HOURS of OPERATION

All listings in the various sections of this book were cross-checked for accuracy. Prices mentioned in the features are subject to change due to fluctuations in the economy and management. Operating hours are also subject to change, especially on a seasonal basis in rural areas. As a rule of thumb, room rates usually increase $5 - $10 per room per year. However because of the high demand for coastal lodging, a feeding frenzy has occurred with excessive (just plain greedy) prices to make up for lost time and money. Rates have sky rocketed and the workers who support these establishments have suffered. People do not forget and corrections in real money and karma are inevitable. Menu prices usually increase about 10% to 20% per year due to inflation and cost of operation. The following price rating symbols accompany each restaurant and lodge.

($) Inexpensive to Moderate: Meals under $15, Lodging $35-$85/2
($$) Moderate to Expensive: Meals $16-$35, Lodging $95-$200/2
($$$) Very Expensive: Meals over $35, Lodging over $200/2

A WORD ABOUT THE REVIEWS

I live here. Since 1975 I have sold over 100,000 guidebooks generating millions of dollars flowing into the north coast economy. I frequent the Mendocino County coastline, wine country, redwoods and mountains. The roads and the people who live here are well known to me and the reviews are accurately written with a depth of first hand experience few travel writers ever achieve. Shop and compare. A color photograph is worth a thousand words. Guide book readers are extremely visually oriented. So, this book is for you.

Each restaurant, accommodation, general store and winery has been personally inspected and the proprietors interviewed. Each restaurant has been dined at prior to being written up. I personally inspect each accommodation. I hope you find what you are looking for.

A WORD OF CAUTION

In the 1970's President Reagan gave the mentally ill bus tickets to two cities in northern California - Bolinas and Mendocino. Combined with a social welfare conveyor belt and progressive liberal tolerance; we have a loose population of undisciplined deviates. Lock your car, protect your loved ones and your pets while visiting Fort Bragg and Mendocino.

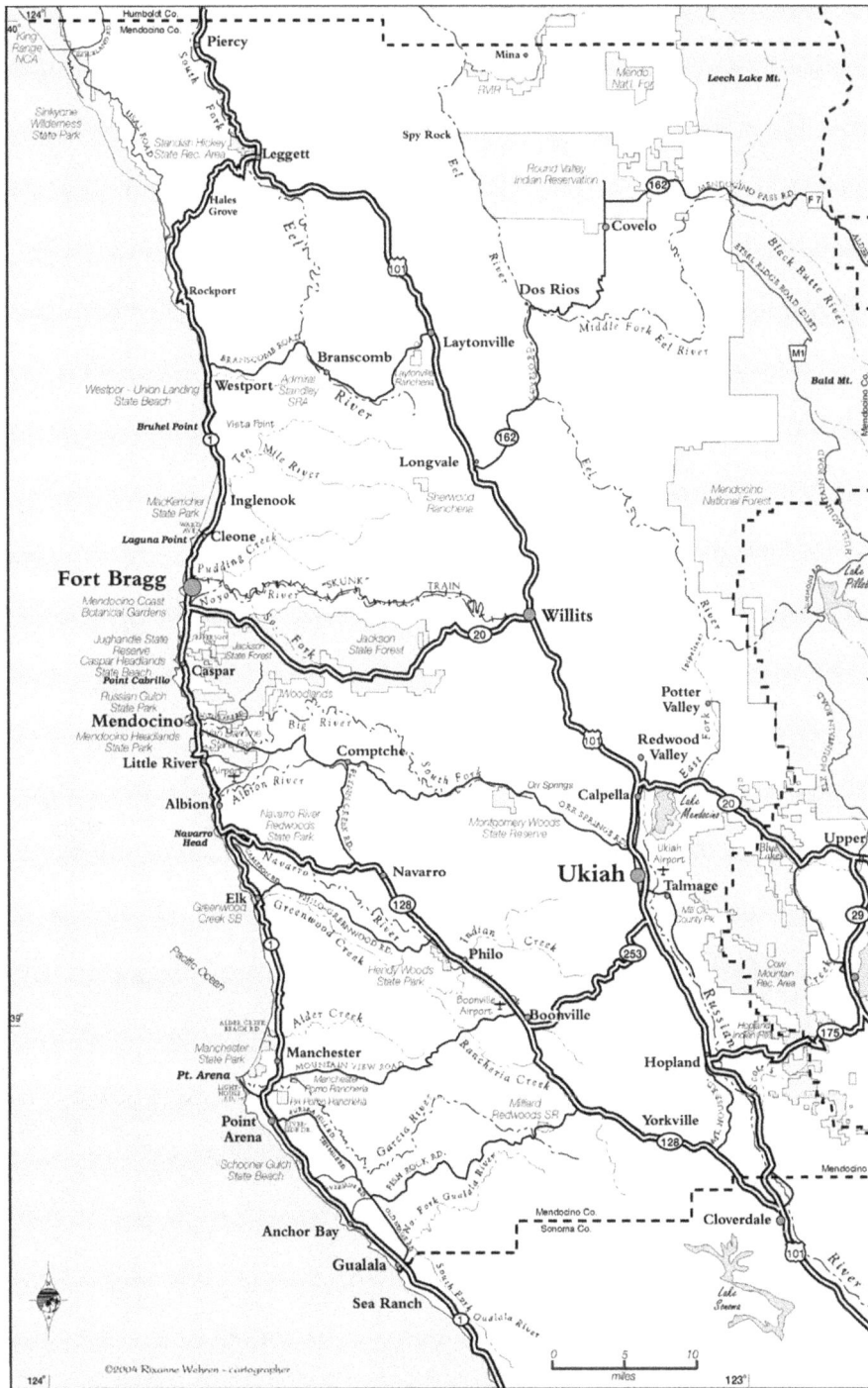

124°
40°
King Range NCA

Humbolt Co.
Mendocino Co.

Piercy

Sinkyone Wilderness State Park

Mina

Mendo. Nat'l For.

Leech Lake Mt.

Round Valley Indian Reservation

Spy Rock

162

Standish Hickey State Rec. Area

Leggett

Hales Grove

Covelo

Rockport

Dos Rios

101

Branscomb

Laytonville

Middle Fork Eel River

Westport

Admiral Standley SRA

Laytonville Rancheria

Westport - Union Landing State Beach

Bald Mt.

Mendocino Co.

Bruhel Point

Vista Point

162

Ten Mile River

Longvale

Mendocino National Forest

MacKerricher State Park

Inglenook

Sherwood Rancheria

Laguna Point

Cleone

Pudding Creek

Lake Pillsb

Fort Bragg

Mendocino Coast Botanical Gardens

SKUNK TRAIN

Willits

Jughandle State Reserve
Caspar Headlands State Beach
Point Cabrillo

Jackson State Forest

Jackson State Forest

20

Russian Gulch State Park

Caspar

Woodlands

Potter Valley

Mendocino

Mendocino Headlands State Park

Big River

101

Redwood Valley

Little River

Comptche

South Fork

Or. Springs

Calpella

Lake Mendocino

20

Albion

Albion River

Navarro River Redwoods State Park

Montgomery Woods State Reserve

Ukiah Airport

Upper

Navarro Head

Navarro

Ukiah

Talmage

29

Elk
Greenwood Creek SB

128

Greenwood Creek

Hendy Woods State Park

Philo

Indian Creek

253

Russian River

175

Pacific Ocean

Alder Creek

Boonville Airport

Boonville

Manchester State Park

Manchester

Mountain View Road

Rancheria Creek

Hopland

Pt. Arena

Manchester Pomo Rancheria

Garcia River

Milliard Redwoods SR

Point Arena

Yorkville

Schooner Gulch State Beach

128

Mendocino

Anchor Bay

Fish Rock Road

North Fork Gualala River

Mendocino Co.
Sonoma Co.

Cloverdale

101

Gualala

Sea Ranch

South Fork Gualala River

Lake Sonoma

River

0   5   10
miles

123°

124°

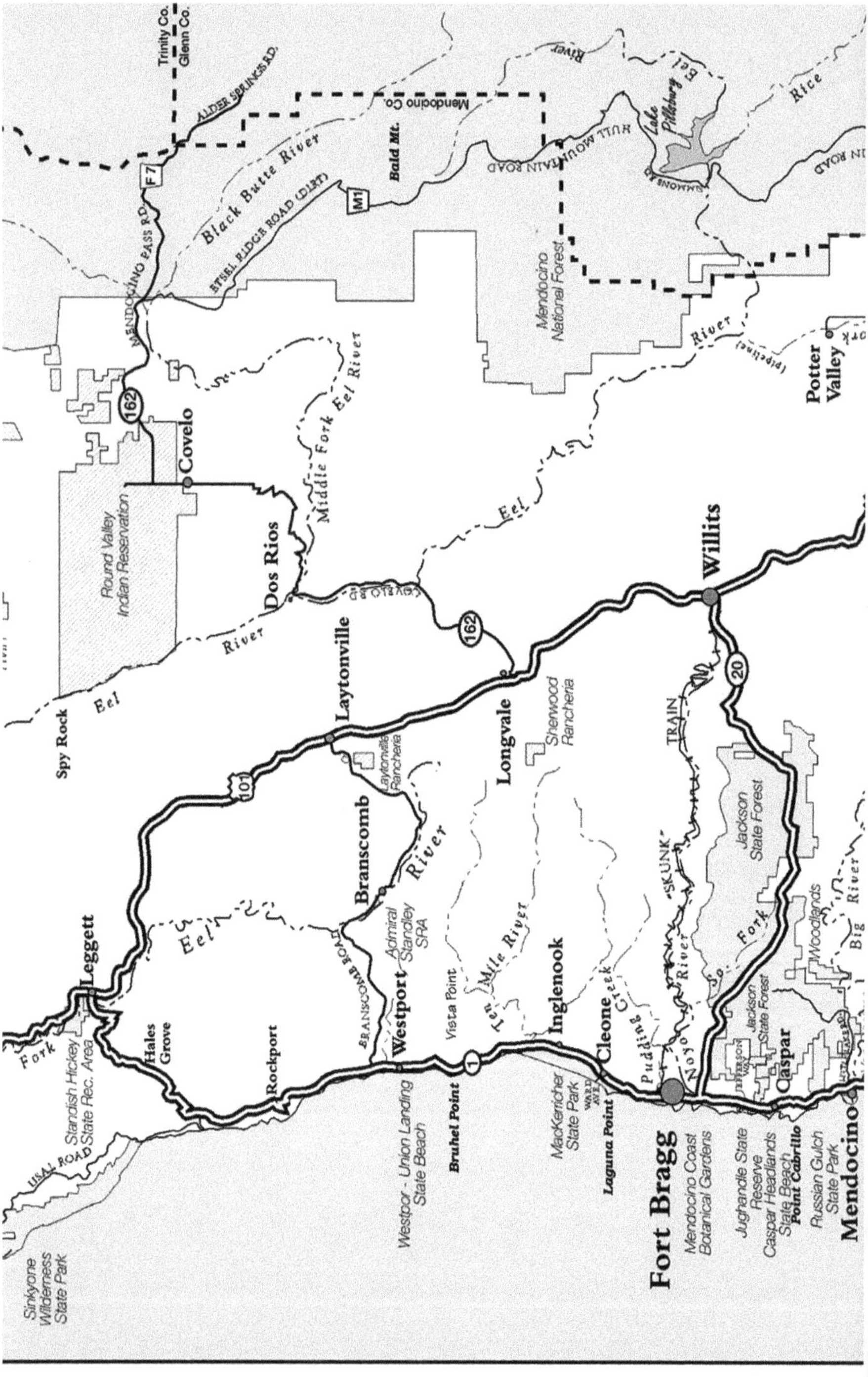

Trinity Co.
Glenn Co.
Mendocino Co.
ALDER SPRINGS RD.
Black Butte River
ETSEL RIDGE ROAD (DIRT)
MENDOCINO PASS RD.
F7
M1
Bald Mt.
HULL MOUNTAIN ROAD
Lake Pillsbury
Eel
River
Rice
SIMMONS RD.
Mendocino National Forest
162
Covelo
Round Valley Indian Reservation
Middle Fork Eel River
Dos Rios
COVELO RD
River
Eel
Potter Valley
Spy Rock
Eel
River
Laytonville
Laytonville Rancheria
Longvale
Sherwood Rancheria
Willits
20
101
Branscomb
River
TRAIN
"SKUNK"
Jackson State Forest
Leggett
Eel
Admiral Standley SRA
Ten Mile River
Inglenook
Big River
Woodlands
Fork
So. Fork
Noyo River
Pudding Creek
Cleone
Hales Grove
Rockport
BRANSCOMB ROAD
Westport
Vista Point
Fork
Standish Hickey State Rec. Area
USAL ROAD
1
Westport - Union Landing State Beach
Bruhel Point
MacKerricher State Park
Laguna Point
Fort Bragg
Mendocino Coast Botanical Gardens
Jackson State Forest
Caspar
Jughandle State Reserve
Caspar Headlands State Beach
Point Cabrillo
Russian Gulch State Park
Mendocino
Sinkyone Wilderness State Park

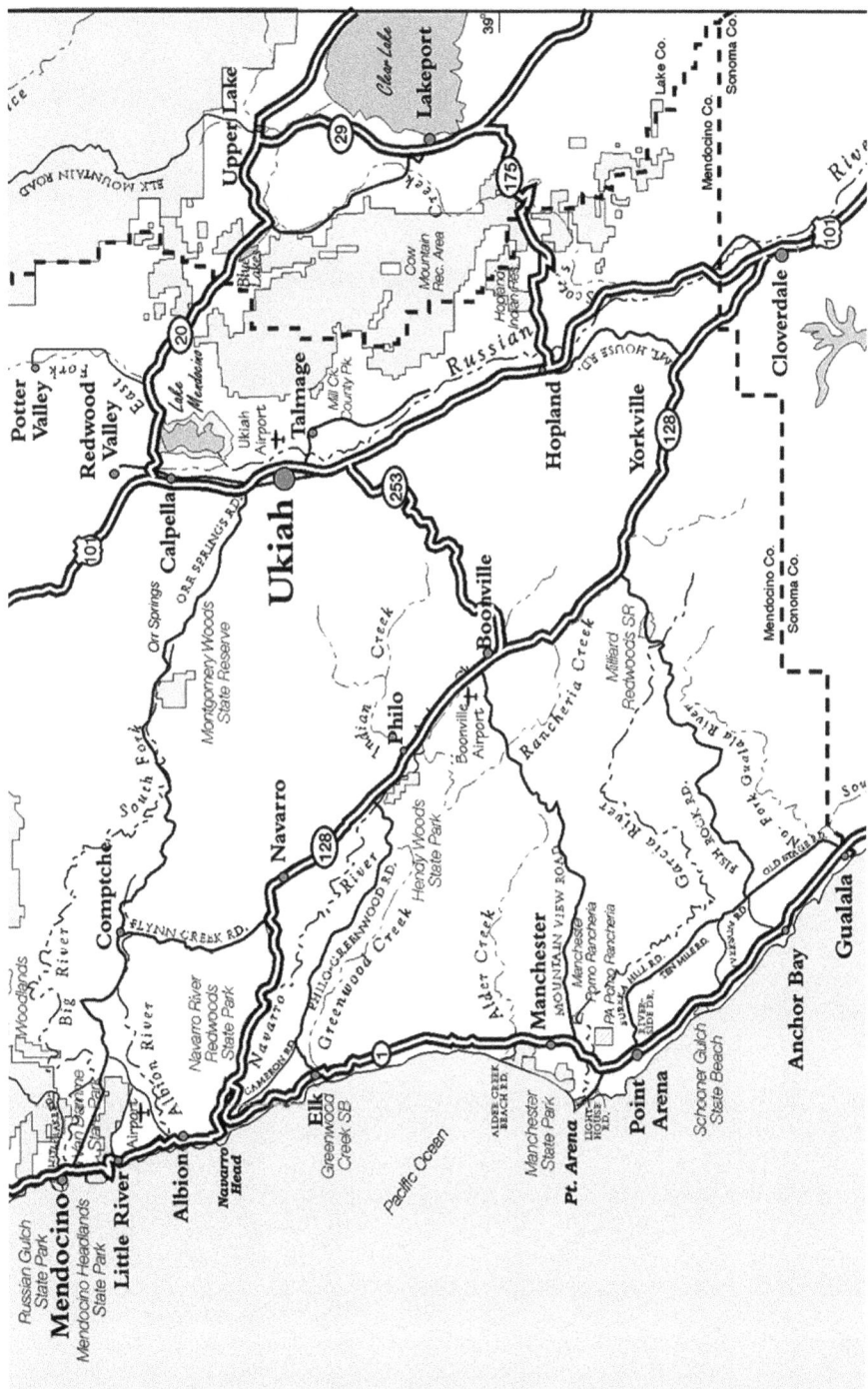

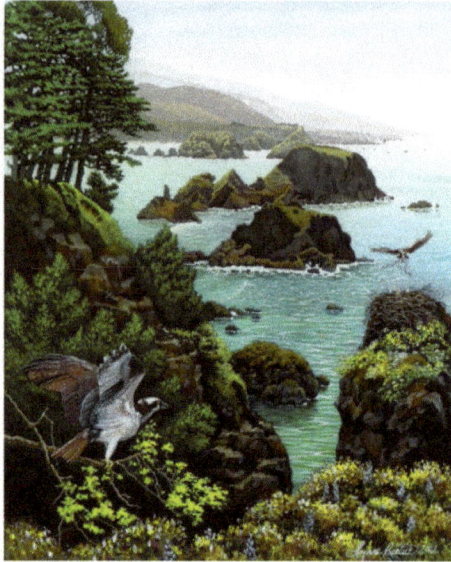

Elk, also known as Greenwood was a lumber port at the turn of the century. This tiny community is perched on the cliffs above the Pacific overlooking rocky coves and sandy beaches. Many find it very healing here as well as an ideal place to re-create! Restaurants, lodging, the healing arts and the great outdoors are all present. Locals state that "It's always a great day in Elk!"

"Room With A View" Painting by Lynne Prentice of Prentice Fine Art Gallery & Framing (707) 937-5205

THE ELK COAST: Manchester, Irish Beach & Elk

MANCHESTER to ELK DINER'S CHOICE: Tele Area Code is (707)
Elk Cove Inn ($$-$$$) 6300 S. Hwy 1, Elk 877-3321 / 800-275-2967;
Elk House ($-$$) 5920 S. Hwy 1 877-3422; **Elk Store** ($-$$) 6101 S
Hwy 1 877-3544; **Greenwood Cafe** ($$) 5928 S. Hwy 1 877-3422;
Harbor House ($$-$$$) 5600 S. Hwy 1 877-3203

MANCHESTER to ELK LODGING:
Elk Cove Inn ($$-$$$) 6300 S. Hwy 1, Elk 877-3321 / 800-275-2967;
Elk Guest House ($$) 5910 S. Hwy 1 877-3422; **Harbor House** ($$-
$$$) 5600 S. Hwy 1 877-3203; **Irish Beach Vacation Homes** ($$-$$$)
Box 337, Manchester, CA. 95459 (707) 882-2467; **Manchester Beach
KOA** ($) Hwy 1 & Kinney Rd. 800-562-4188; **Sacred Rock Inn** ($$-
$$$) 5928 S. Hwy 1 877-3422; **Victorian Garden Inn** ($$) 14409 S.
Hwy 1, Manchester 882-3606.

TOURIST INFO, GENERAL STORES, GIFTSHOPS and the ARTS:
Elk Store ($-$$) 6101 S Hwy 1 877-3411; **Elk Studio Galley** ($-$$$)
6031 S. Hwy 1 877-1128; **Matson's Merchantile** ($-$$) 6061 S. Hwy
1, **S&B Market** ($-$$) 19400 S. Hwy 1 882-2805.
TOWING and GENERAL AUTO REPAIR: Elk Garage ($-$$$) 6061
Hwy 1, Elk 1-800-483-3444   AAA - 24 Hour Towing and Emergencies.
HEALING ARTS and the GREAT OUTDOORS:
Body Works ($$) 877-3430; **Elk Studio of Healing Arts** ($$) 6147 S
Hwy 1, 877-3505; **Ross Ranch Horseback Riding** ($$) 877-1834.

ELK COVE INN, RESTAURANT and SPA

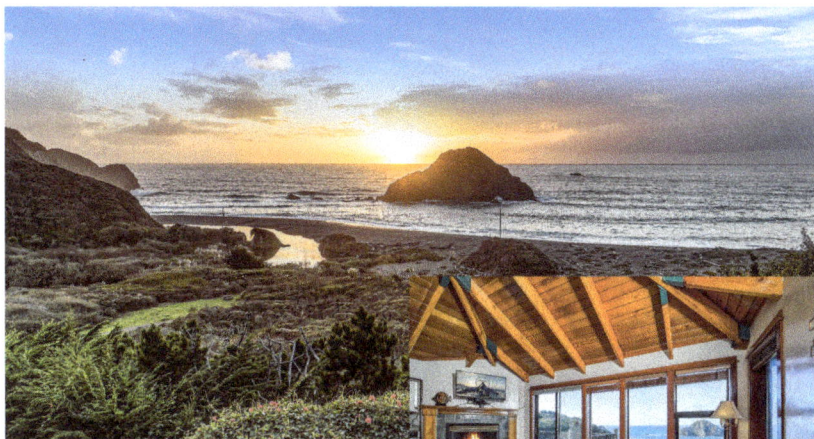

The Elk Cove Inn and Spa is a small family run historical Inn with sixteen unique and beautiful rooms, and an unpretentious welcoming atmosphere that makes every guest feel like family. A rarity on the Mendocino Coast, this Inn boasts direct beach access to Greenwood State Beach, which can be seen from any of our ocean-view rooms.

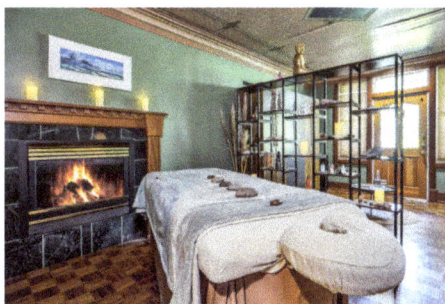

The Inn also offers all the necessary amenities so you may kick back, relax and just take the time to be present. Spa services, a bountiful breakfast delivered in-room, exceptional dinners at Sibo, the on premises restaurant as well as different add-ons can make your stay even more memorable and are all available upon request.

The Elk Cove Inn is also pet friendly, Melissa and Victor, property owners have pets of their own and know all about traveling with pets. Your dog will be able to take walks on Greenwood State beach with you and will receive their own welcome basket when you arrive. For convenience, we offer in-room dining so they won't feel left behind at dinner time. The staff and setting are magical and this can very well become one of your most memorable vacations.

$$-$$$ ELK COVE INN

Breakfast, Dinner, Lodging & Spa
on the Spectacular Mendocino Coast
6300 S. Highway One, Elk, CA.
https://elkcoveinn.com
Reservations 1-800-275-2967
1-707-877-3321

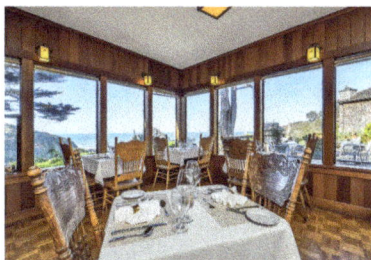

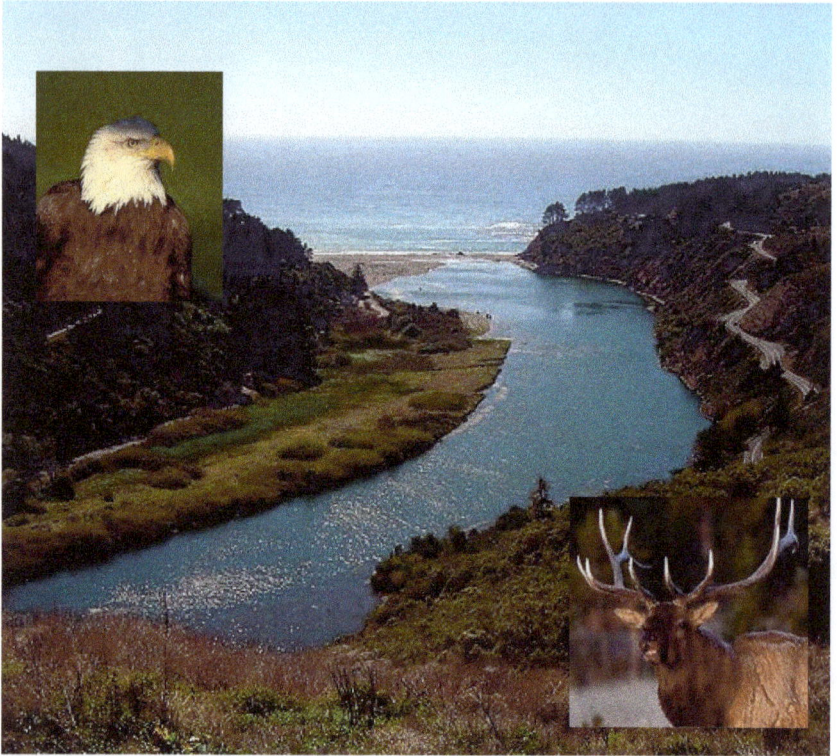

NAVARRO RIVER STATE BEACH

Navarro Beach Campground is the best of all waterside worlds. Fall asleep to ocean songs. Be a neighbor to swimming holes and translucent river currents. Inhale the fresh bite of salt and forest. Cherish views of truly jaw dropping sunsets and partake in the joys of a small scale campground where you can adequately remove yourself from overpopulation anxiety. This beach campground sits beside a stretch of driftwood scattered sand that adjoins the mouth of the Navarro River. Navarro provides a concise 10 site spot and you stake your claim via the more classic first-come first-served approach. This means - plan to grab your spot early and don't wait to pull in at 11pm with no back up plan. Bring layers, but expect summer heat that differs from the normal coastal camping experience and enjoy the payoff of being close to so much skin cooling, soul warming water. The sweet canopy of second growth redwood giants is a stroll away. Be aware both preditor and prey walk this beach by day and night. Protect your loved ones - both two legged and four legged. Rangers and life guards can arrive in minutes.

$ NAVARRO RIVER STATE BEACH   Box 440, Mendocino, CA. 95460
Ocean & Riverview Camping / No Showers, Danger - River mouth hazardous
https://www.parks.ca.gov/?page_id=435   Park Brochure (Link Below)
https://www.parks.ca.gov/pages/435/files/NavarroRiverRedwoodsWeb2011.pdf
Overnight Camping - 1 vehicle $45/night 1-800-444-PARK /(707) 937-5804
Drop - Ins or Reservations at   http://www.reservecalifornia.com

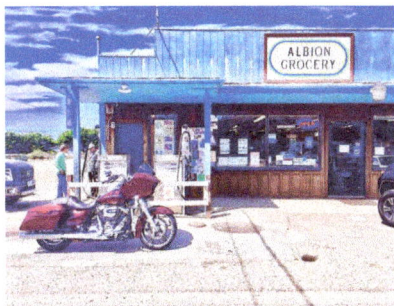

ALBION STORE

The Albion Grocery is a great supply center for explorers of the Mendocino Coast. This spacious grocery store is under the ownership of Prabhleen Singh and Navjeet Kaur. In the gourmet deli an assortment of home-made salads, sandwiches, International dishes and health food with all the necessities for an afternoon picnic or vacation home or RV meal are showcased. Fresh coffee and espressos are made from organic beans. Camping and outdoor cooking equipment, bait and tackle, nautical gear and firewood are among the on-going list of supplies stocked for the great outdoors. The wine selection represents Mendocino's finest wineries. Gasoline and motor oil is also sold. Next door is the Albion Post Office, and a hardware store and down in the harbor are campgrounds, RV parks, boat launching facilities, a laundromat and excellent bird watching.

$-$$ ALBION MARKET   *Box 280, Base of Albion Ridge,*
General Store, Deli, Propane & Gas Station   *Albion, CA. 95410*
Open daily 7am - 6pm   *(707) 937-5784 Information*

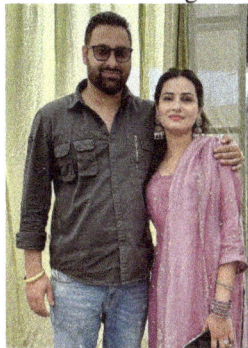

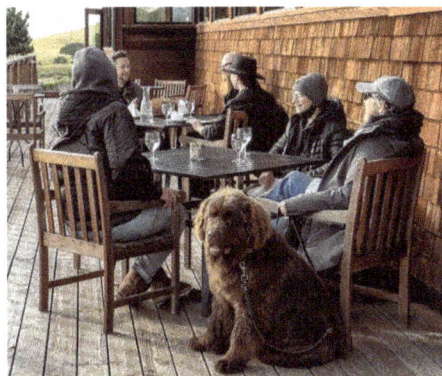

LEDFORD HOUSE

A favorite, with a long history, this seaside restaurant with lofty cliffside views of the crashing surf is one of Mendocino's finest restaurants. Owner/chefs Tony & Lisa Geer create inspiring and romantic dinners. Comforting soups and garden fresh salads (garnished with flowers) are a work of art. Bistro dishes (from $25) and dinners (served a la carte with fresh vegetables from $35) include fresh fish stew in white wine, tomato, fennel and saffron broth with Crostini and Aioli, potato Ginocchi with gorgonzola, and pan seared wild king salmon. The wine list, sumptuous desserts, crackling fire and view make for exceptional memories.

$$ THE LEDFORD HOUSE   *3000 North Hwy 1, Albion, CA. 95410*
Bistro French / Hints of Basque   *Dinners from 5pm Wed - Sun*
Seasonal Sun. Brunch. 9am - 2pm   *(707) 937-0282 Res. advised*
Located west of Hwy 1 at base of Albion Ridge   *http://www.ledfordhouse.com/*

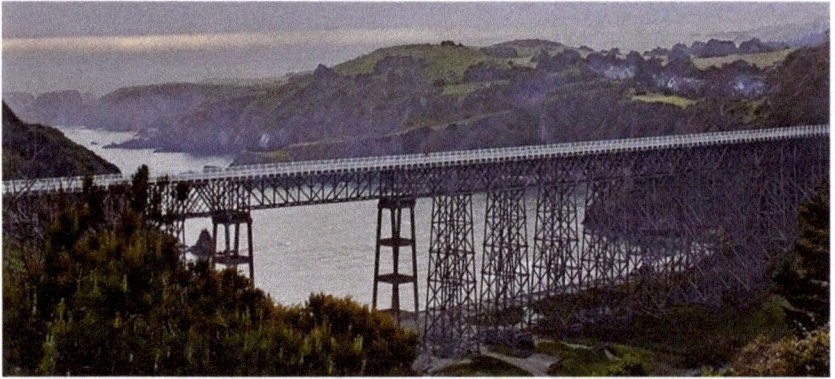

The historic 970 foot long Albion River Bridge was built in 1944 and is the only remaining wooden bridge on California State Route 1. A new earthquake / tsunami safe bridge is scheduled to be built next to the orginal bridge at some time in the future. RV Camping, fishing, birdwatching, lodging and dining are nearby.

ALBION RIVER CAMPGROUND and MARINA

Beneath the Albion River Bridge on a broad river valley flat is the Albion River Fishing Village and Campground. Available for big groups and open camping, the fees vary for tent or car camping, $50 for water, wifi and electricity and $60 for full RV hook-ups ($5 day use and $2 per dog). There are hot showers and bathrooms. Schooner's Landing Selkie Cove Campground is just up river and is a membership only "Eco Club".

$-$$ ALBION RIVER CAMPGROUND   Base of Albion Ridge, Albion, CA.
Camping, Store, RV Hook-Ups, Showers, Bird Watching, Kayaking, Fishing
Open daily 8am - 4pm http://www.albionrivercampground.com (707) 937-0606
$$ SCHOONER'S LANDING   P.O. Box 613, Albion, CA 95410
https://www.schoonerslanding-albion.com/   (707) 937-5707

TERRA MAR RESTAURANT and MENDOCINO INN

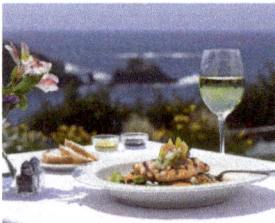

The Albion River Inn and Restaurant is now the Terra Mar Restaurant and Mendoino Coast Inn which is owned by SCP Lodging out of Los Angelos. 22 luxurious cliffside oceanview rooms feature fireplaces, decks, and spa-tubs. Rates range from $215 to $438 /2 per night, and include a full breakfast served in the restaurant each morning.

Terra Mar Restaurant is open for breakfast and dinner. The menu features an array of fresh seafood, locally sourced produce and proteins, wild mushrooms, creative pasta dishes, and heavenly desserts. For current PDFs of the breakfast and dinner menu visit their website. Chef Kenny Boyle believes "that great food starts with great ingredients."

$$-$$$ TERRA   MAR   RESTAURANT   and   MENDOCINO   INN
Oceanview Lodging, Dining, Full Bar   3790 N. Hwy 1, Albion, CA. 95410
Fresh Seafood & Coastal Cuisine, Full Bar, numerous amenities, fireplaces & spas
https://scphotel.com/mendocino-coast/food-drink/albion-river-inn-restaurant/
(707) 937-1919 Dinner Reservations   (800) 479-7944 in Northern California

The ANDIRON - SEASIDE INN & CABINS

Everybody is looking for a cozy little cabin love nest with forest and ocean views on the Mendocino Coast. Such is what you will find at the Andiron Seaside Inn and Cabins just south of Little River.

Your friendly owners, Scott Connolly and Madeline Stanionis state, "we love our cabins and rooms and hope you do too! Our inn was built in 1959, with the cabins spread out over five acres of meadow and woods. Every single cabin and room is entirely unique, and furnished with salvage, and rehabbed furniture and furnishings. You'll find all kinds of fun and funky touches, like: vintage Viewmasters, unusual mid-century lamps, large wall murals, and classic games and puzzles. Also all the practical things are covered too: each has a deck, private bathroom, TV/DVD player, refrigerator, barbecue, and coffee maker." Many rooms have kitchenettes and most have fireplaces (rates are from $149 - $300). Additionally, our weekend Happy Hours feature Cannabis and Hemp cocktails. The cabins also share a magical hot tub in the woods. Andiron is pet friendly.

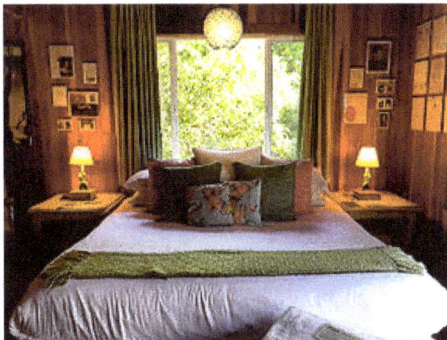

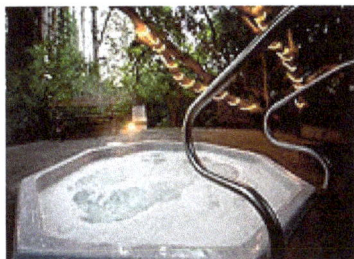

$$ ANDIRON SEASIDE INN & CABINS   *6051 N. Hwy 1, Little River, CA.*
Cozy Oceanview Cabins   *https://www.theandiron.com/*
Credit / Debit Cards   (707) 937-1543   or 1-800-955-MIST (6478) Res. Sug.

WOOD HAVEN

Wood haven is located on Pegasus Farm, a rural organic farm near Mendocino California. Your accommodations are loaded with rare and exotic hand crafted redwood heartwood. Amenities include a full gourmet kitchen, bath, loft with double bed, double bed downstairs and a wood stove for heat.

Explore the beautiful gardens, the magical redwood fairy ring and pond out back. Lounge in the meadow and take a moment of zen, or start a fire in the yard lounge. Star watch at night. Do yoga in the grassy meadow, play from the various instruments in the main farm house. The options go on and on....... and Mendocino is but a short drive to the north.

$$ WOOD HAVEN at PEGASUS FARM   *Little River Road, Little River, CA.*
Cozy Cabin on an Organic Farm   *(707) 937-2746 Reservations Necessary*

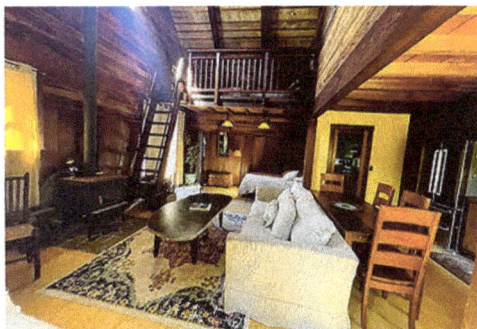

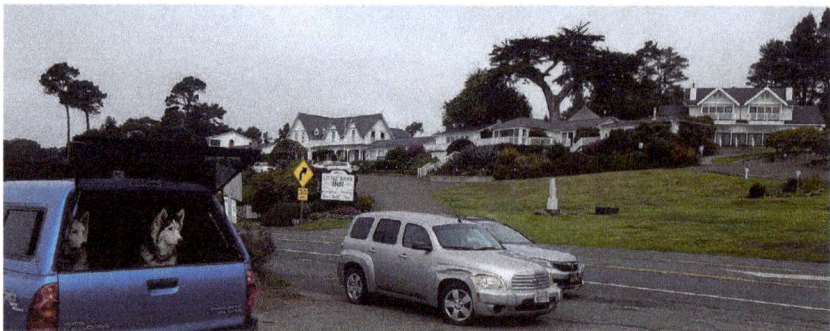

Dark moody winter skies approach as locals check their mail and shop at the Little River Market. Hilltop are the cozy fireplaces, libations and comfort food of Little River Inn.

LITTLE RIVER INN

There is quite a selection of accommodations to choose from at Little River Inn. In the historic Inn (circa 1853) are Victorian rooms with commanding views overlooking Van Damme Cove with its surf-tossed rock outcroppings. To the north, nestled into the hillside, are two-story rooms that open out onto spacious balcony walk-ways with sweeping ocean views. To the south, amid the meandering gardens, are a variety of units, each with a commanding view of the seascape, a cozy woodburning fireplace, and some have a two-person luxury tubs. Massages or body treatments are on-site in the day spa and guests can also enjoy a round of golf followed by a feast in the Little River dining room's garden setting. Entree ingredients come from Mendocino county farms and ranches, seafood from Noyo Harbor and vegetables harvested from local gardens. Ole's Whale Watch Bar, open nightly, serves cocktails and a bar menu. Room service is offered from both the dining room and bar.

$$-$$$LITTLE RIVER INN   *Hwy 1, Little River, California 95456*
Dinner - Lodging   Tennis Courts & Golf Course,   (707) 937-5667
Dinner: Sun.-Thurs. 6-8:30pm; Fri. and Sat. 6-9pm.   http://www.littleriverinn.com
Breakfast & SundayBrunch Full Bar & Restaurant 1-888-INN-LOVE (466-5683) Res.

LITTLE RIVER MARKET

The Little River Market is located 2 miles south of Mendocino on the ocean side of Route 1. Here north coast visitors can pull off the road to gas up or make a phone call and then go inside and browse the shelves of this exceptional gourmet general store and market. In the deli you can purchase delicious homemade sandwiches, meatloaf, smoked salmon, deviled eggs and a variety of salads. Enjoy the fabulous picture window views of the sea while snacking. Shy proprietor Young Ji and staff have always preferred stocking higher quality brands and locally made organic goodies. A very nice variety of craft beers and California vintage wines are also carried plus fresh brewed organic coffee.

$-$$ LITTLE RIVER MARKET   *7746 Hwy 1, Little River, CA 95456*
General Store, Deli, & Gas Station   Open daily 8am - 6pm   (707) 937-5133

HERITAGE HOUSE

One of the most famous destinations on the Mendocino Coast is the Heritage House, located just south of Little River. In 1949 Lauren and Hazel Dennen purchased the property and began creating Mendocino's first country inn. Film stars Alan Alda and Ellen Burstyn brought new meaning to aging gracefully by arriving as young lovers and returning as grandparents in the motion picture "Same Time Next Year;" filmed on location in 1971.

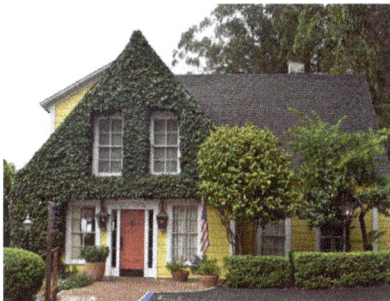

Today the Heritage House is owned by a billionaire and his management group. A lot has been lost since the days the Dennens greeted guests and local business people with kindness and appreciation. Sixty nine cottages, rooms and suites are scattered over 37 acres of gardens along the rugged Pacific coastline. The Heritage House Resort also features a spa to soothe aching muscles. The restaurant and full bar offers breakfast, lunch and dinners.

$$-$$$ HERITAGE HOUSE

Restaurant, Gardens, Lodging, Spa   5200 N. Hwy 1, Little River, CA. 95456
https://www.heritagehouseinn.com   Front Desk Reservations 707-202-9000

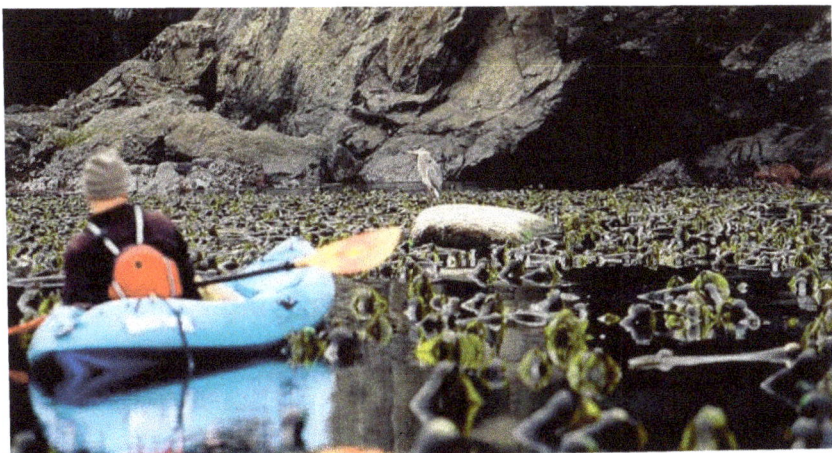

Champion surfer and expert ocean kayaker, Craig Comen, leads small groups of adventurers on seasonal tours from Van Damme State Park just to the north. You can contact Craig at his Kayak Mendocino website at http://www.kayakmendocino.com

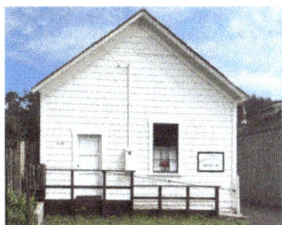

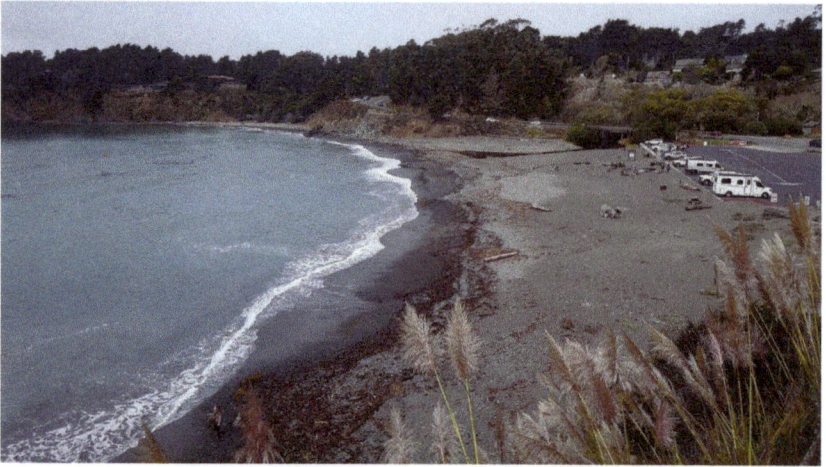

VAN DAMME STATE PARK and BEACH

If people are acting crazy or the stress of the day has gotten to you then drive through or walk slowly along fern lined Little River under the coastal forest canopy of Van Damme State Park. Take it all in - slowly. . . n listen to the breeze rustle the leaves and the distant ocean waves. Steelhead hide in the dark pools, owls hoot at night beneath a heavenly tapestry of stars. Here, humankind, the caretaker, has fulfilled their godly task and preserved a beautiful natural setting to relax and rejuvenate in. There are 74 tent or car/RV campsites with water and picnic tables (no electricity - bring portable solar panels). Rates are $45 / night which includes one vehicle (additional vehicle $10), day use $8,

$ VAN DAMME STATE BEACH   *Box 440, Mendocino, CA. 95460*
Forest Camping, Hot Showers, Fire Pits, Oceanview & Beach, Kayaking
https://www.parks.ca.gov/?page_id=433   Park Brochure (Link Below)
PARK MAP: https://www.parks.ca.gov/pages/433/files/VanDamSBPDF.pdf
http://www.reservecalifornia.com   1-800-444-PARK (7275) /(707) 937-5804

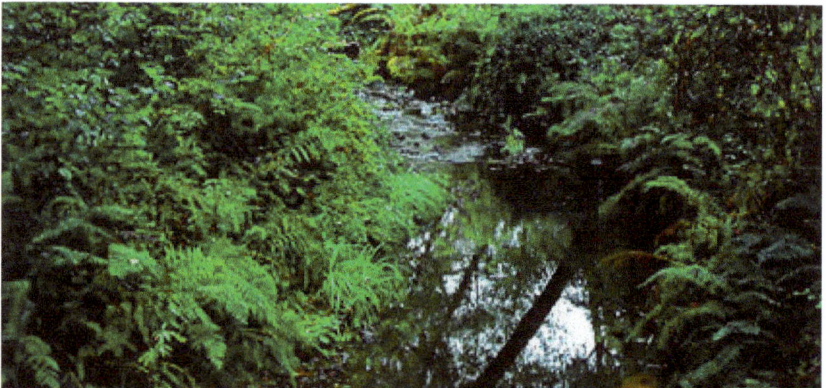

SOUL COMMUNITY PLANET MENDOCINO INN and FARM

The Soul Community Planet (SCP) Mendocino Inn and Farm is comprised of six buildings and a cottage which occupies fifteen rolling acres of woodland, pastures, and gardens. Rates vary seasonal and depend on what day of the week you stay and vary from $194 to $340 / 2 per night. There are special AAA, AARP and government rates. Pet dogs can stay for $35 per night. A homemade breakfast of juice, fruit, muffins and egg shuffles is delivered to your door the following morning. Amenities are numerous and include fireplaces, a spa, fitness center, internet access, meeting facilities and catering of events with 31 rooms, some offering avocado mattresses, luxurious bedding, and forest or ocean views. A flock of chickens provide fresh organic eggs and llamas you can visit gently graze in the meadow.

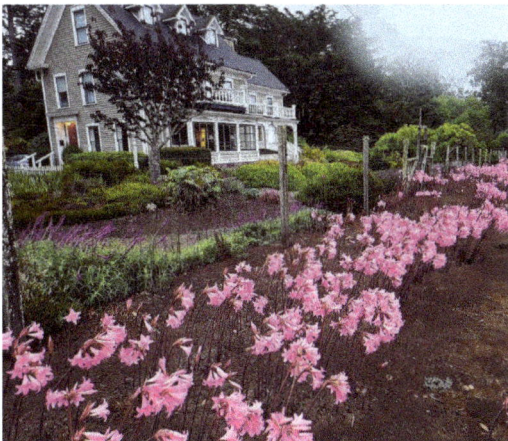

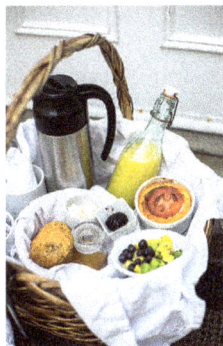

The owners state "Every time you choose to stay at an SCP hotel, you are consciously choosing to join a community that is driving positive change in the world around us." A look at the non-profits and causes on their website reveals this portion of the money you pay for lodging is shipped out of the area. This is a growing concern on the part of many on the Mendocino Coast. There are only a few locally owned mom n pop lodging facilities left on the coast. In addition *LOCAL* veteran and senior citizen needs seem to be ignored.

The Lodge ($224 - $270/2) is located among the gardens offering guest rooms with large windows to enjoy views of the surrounding greenery. The stately and historic 1867 Farmhouse ($243 - $287/2) offers coastline views. The Cobbler's House ($194 - $225/2), offers two common spaces on the main floor, along with five guest rooms and suites. Designed on three-levels, the Fourequarters Building offers four guest rooms, all with a fireplace, and an outdoor seating area for guests. The Stevenscroft Building ($232 - $260/2) provides a private entrance to each of the four guest rooms and is nestled between the llama pastures and organic garden. The Carriage House King Loft ($232 - $260/2) is a bright and spacious suite with two fireplaces. This is a flawed but remarkable destination with lots of choices.

$$-$$$ SPC MENDOCINO INN and FARM - formally GLENDEVEN
Bed & Breakfast Farm   8211 N. Hwy 1, Little River, CA 95456 (707) 937-0083
https://www.https://scphotel.com/mendocino/rooms/   1-800-822-4536 Reserve

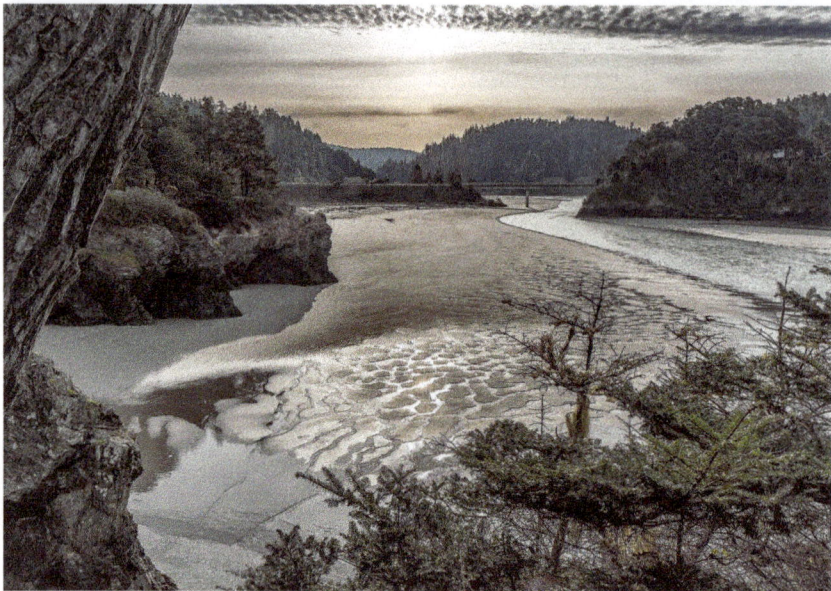

BIG RIVER BEACH and ESTERO at LOW TIDE

You can spend hours at Big River Beach and Estero just watching the ebb and flow of the salt water meeting the fresh water of the river. The colors are constantly changing and you never know who you are going to meet. Some visitors and their dogs are friendly, some are not. Some build campfires and spend the night propped up against a driftwood log wind-break to keep warm. A hot cup of coffee or meal is just up the cliff in Mendocino. No doubt solutions to problems in your life come to you and probably more than one proposal has been made at sunset. The resultant couple return years later with their children to start the cycle of life all over again. The above photograph, "Luminous Morning," was created by Scott Chieffo of the Mendocino Coast Photography Gallery. You can view his work and contact him at https://www.schieffophotography.com

MENDOCINO GROVE

The secluded entrance to Mendocino Grove just south of Mendocino on State Highway 1 is very inviting. Entering and exiting the main entrance is dangerous as vehicles whip up and down this stretch of Hwy 1 with it's blind curves. Drive up to the top of the hillside and you get your first glimpse of what appears to be a yuppie FEMA camp with all manner of liberal lifestyles and refugees. Check in at the concierge tent and tour to your tent site. This enchanting forest setting is a natural sanctuary from the stresses of life. Here you can bask in the healing energy of Mendocino Grove with its distant views of Mendocino Bay. There are over 30 comfortable tent sites, with hot shower spa, dog park and hiking trails. Mendocino with its galleries, restaurants and marijuana dispensaries is just to the north; past the lookout where the Park Rangers and CHP keep watch.

$$-$$$ MENDOCINO GROVE   *9601 N. Hwy. 1, Mendocino, Ca 95460*
HIP CAMPING, Forest Bathing, Dog Park, Group Meetings, Oceanviews
http://www.mendocinogrove.com   *(707) 880-7710 Reservations Advised*

STANFORD INN by the SEA and RAVEN'S RESTAURANT

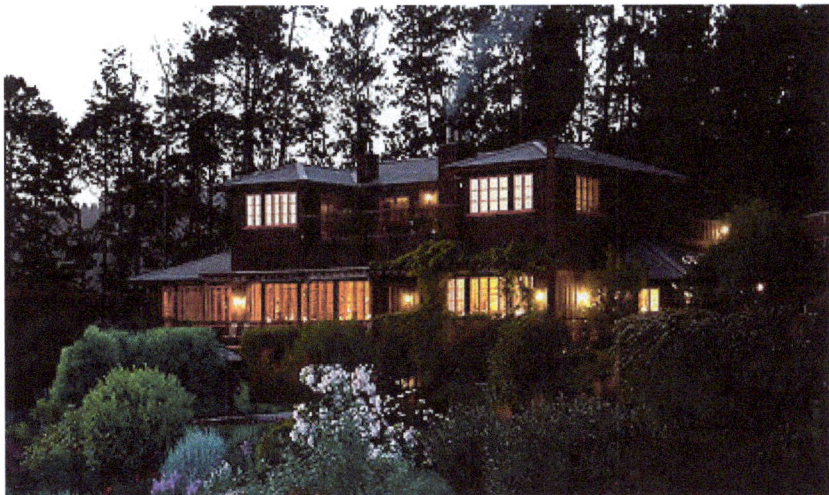

Kind and generous visionaries, Jeff and Joan Stanford have pioneered many healthy trends in Mendocino County. They have created a world class vegan-vegetarian restaurant, promoted alternative health care and diet, are home to large organic gardens co-created with John Jeavons, and Matt Drewno complete with heirloom seed bank of non-GMO varieties, built a large indoor garden swimming pool, and purchased a fleet of kayaks and "water world" catamarans for adventures up the Big River estero. Last but not least, they rescued horses, llamas, dogs and cats. You and your children should really enjoy it here.

Each of the rooms are tastefully decorated with comforters and an array of unique antique furnishings and fixtures. All have private baths, televisions, VCR's, coffee makers, telephones, sundecks and toasty fireplaces (from $265/2). A full breakfast is served in the Ravens restaurant with organic produce from the certified organic gardens. You can canoe Big River estuary with the tides and spot osprey and river otter. The lodge is surrounded by thick forests of fern, fir, bull pine, redwood and cypress. Ask about the special mushroom tours and learn about the nueral net in the soil beneath you. More than one life has been touched or transformed after a stay at Stanford Inn by the Sea.

$$-$$$ STANFORD INN by the SEA   *$-$$ RAVEN'S RESTAURANT*

Oceanview Rooms   *Canoe rentals, fine dining and whale watching.*
*On the Comptche-Ukiah Rd. at Route 1   Over 20 spacious rooms just south of
the Big River Bridge. Finest vegetarian restaurant in Mendocino, Gardens*
Major credit cards   3790 Hwy 1 N., Mendocino, CA 95460
http://www.standordinn.com   800-331-8884 Res. Advised

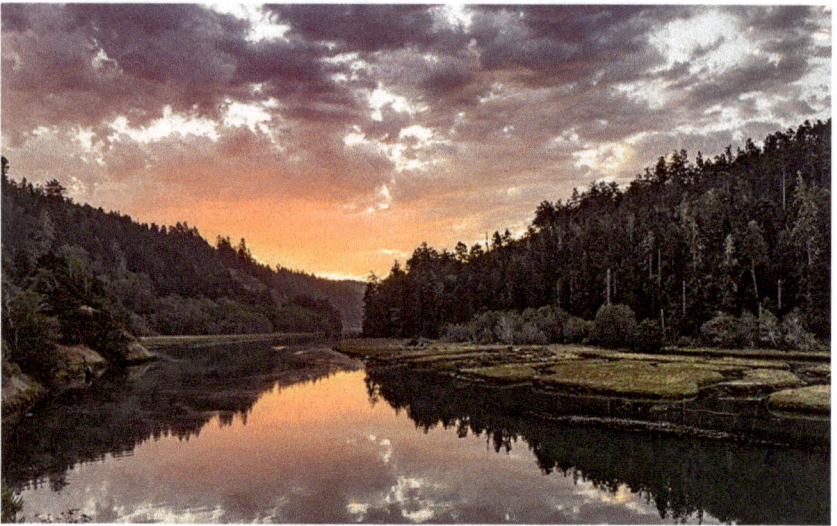

BIG RIVER ESTERO BEACHES, BRIDGE and HIKING TRAILS

MENDOCINO: Historic Victorian Village by the Sea

Mendocino, located 120 miles north of San Francisco, is a coastal village with a "small town personality," which was named by Spanish explorers for Cape Mendocino. The population is 800 plus and Mendocino is on the National Register of Historic Places. It can be reached from the southeast by State Highway 128, from the northeast by State Highway 20, the north/south by state Highway One or by traveling the remote and picturesque Comptche-Ukiah Road. Rarely does the temperature go over 89 degrees, however days can be windy and winter storms fierce and exciting.

The cleanest air and clearest light blesses visitors and the artist community who create here. Visitors escape the summer heat and stay in a multitude of hotels, bed n breakfast inns, state park campgrounds and vacation rental homes. Demand from refugees is high, so realestate is pricey and tight. Lots of places to park your adventure van or RV along the cliffs or in the forests. Keep your vehicle and loved ones (2 n 4 legged) secure during the day and locked at night.

Fancy to traditional restaurants satisfy appetites from raw-vegan to steaks and seafood. Picnics to go, pizza, smoothies, cheese burgers, chili rellenos, smoked salmon, clam chowder, salsa & chips, organic garden fresh salads, cinnamon rolls, mochas and lattes; we have it all. Whether you are looking for economy to extravagant, you will not be disappointed. Lots of historic buildings, galleries and shops to explore. Kayaking, surfing, wildlife watching (people and nature), star watching, beach combing and to the north "big city Fort Bragg" and the remote Lost Coast. Many come here for the inner as well as the outer journey and to heal and reflect. I hope you find what you are looking for.

MENDOCINO: Historic Victorian Village Map

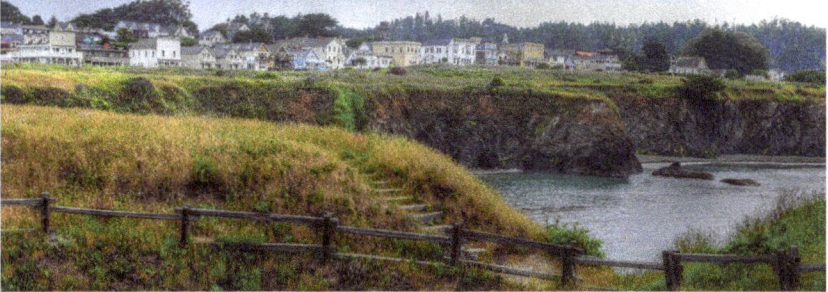

Award winning photographer Russ Christoff took the above photo and named it "Fence and Main". Russ states, "The split rail fence surrounding Mendocino's "blow hole" can be the perfect foreground for the main street. The area is also a great walk with breathtaking views of the bay behind you, and closer to the bluffs can be found a great picnic spot . . . all your own."

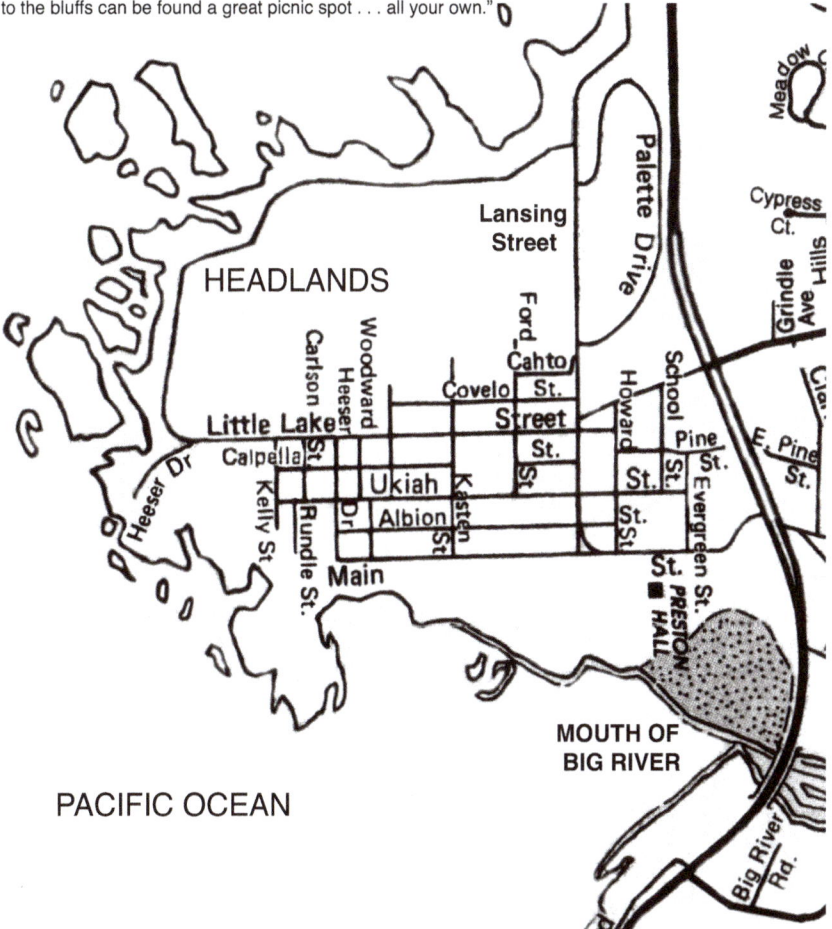

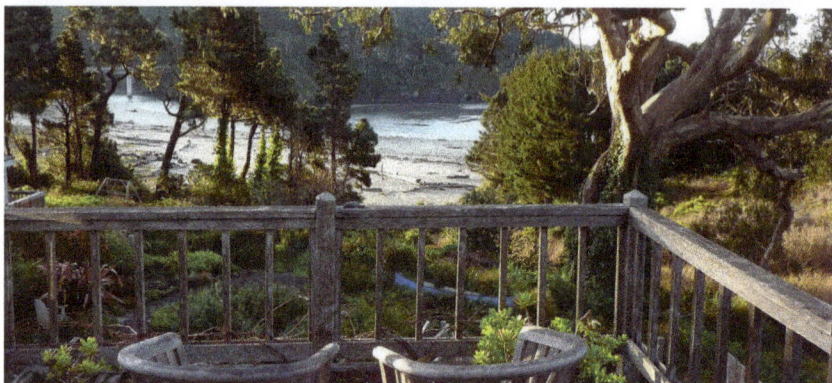

ALEGRIA OCEANFRONT INN and COTTAGES

Algeria is an amazing property set 85 feet up on the Mendocino Headlands with ocean, forest and garden views. It feels good here - energetically and otherwise. Over the last 26 years owners, Elaine and Eric Hillesland, have methodically renovated and improved the inn to make guests feel really comfortable. You can choose from three cottages, eight rooms and suites and three vacation homes with rates from $170 - $500 + for 2 per night. Cottages include the Garden, Driftwood, Tree House, Sea Breeze, Cove Cottage; plus a loft room and village farm retreat setting. The Cove Cottage is the closest accommodation to the water in Mendocino Village. A tansu created just for this space efficiently holds the coffee maker, refrigerator, small microwave oven, and utensils and glassware you need. A Jotul wood stove with glass doors provides a crackling fire, perfect for a romantic evening. Sleeps are deep here.

The following morning a breakfast with fresh fruit, organic juices, teas and coffees are served, as well as hot chocolate. Hot entrees include frittatas, baked egg dishes, pancakes, waffles and locally sourced sausage. Baked goods are always made in-house from scratch. Special diets are gladly accommodated.

$$-$$$ ALEGRIA INN http://www.oceanfrontmagic.com/   (707) 937-5150
Cottages, Rooms and Suites Box 1881, 998 Main St., Mendocino, CA. 95460

SEAGULL INN

The front entrance of this inn is marked by a hand-carved seagull on a large driftwood sign with the words "Seagull Inn — Lodging." First converted to an inn in the 60's, the rooms have provided wonderful shelter for almost 6 decades (rates are $149 - $199). Your innkeeper/ owners are Ian and Kim Roth. There are 3 rooms on the first floor which have been christened the Geranium, Look Out One and Two. On the second floor are the Driftwood (with gas fireplace), Abalone, Sea Urchin and Sand Dollar. The Barn has a double bed loft and stairway with sitting room and queen bed downstairs (ideal for families — sleeps 6). A hearty breakfast is included and served in your room. Beautifully landscaped grounds and flower gardens are outside your window.

$$-$$$ SEAGULL INN   http://www.seagullbb.com   *1-888-937-5204 Toll Free*
Oceanview Bed & Breakfast   *Open all year Call for a free brochure*
44960 Albion St., Mendocino, CA 95460   *(707) 937-5204 Res. Advised*

YOGA and AYURVEDA HEALTH

Yoga, massage therapy, diet and nutrition can add years to your life. Cindy Sims, a Mendocino Yoga teacher, teaches the ancient practice of Ayurveda to promote the health of her patients and students. She has a new studio and private practice and can be reached for current times and locations by visiting her website. Many are happy and have benefited from her expert help and experience .

$$-$$$ YOGA and
AYURVEDA HEALTH with CINDY SIMS
Yoga and Lifestyle Health
Classes are held in Mendocino   *Check Website for Locations and Times*
https://www.cindysims.com/   *(707) 753-0744 Information and Sessions*

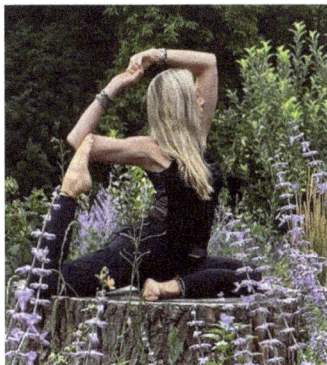

SWEETWATER INN AND ECO SPA

Relaxation and rejuvenation await you at the Sweetwater Gardens Health Spa. Overnight accommodations from $70/2 (pet friendly) and vacation homes (all with hot tubs) from $225/2 are available including luxury oceanview suites, and choice of 3 romantic water tower rooms from $110-$200. Sweethearts never had it so good with expert masseuse's and body-workers on staff, nutritious herb teas and light snacks in the lobby, and choice of private or public hot tub and sauna rooms in this peaceful setting.

$-$$ SWEETWATER INN & HEALTH SPA   *Box 337, 955 Ukiah St.*
Health Retreat, Hot Tubs, Sauna & Massage   *Mendocino, CA. 95460*
Open Mon - Thur. 2pm to 10pm / Fri & Sat noon to 11pm (707) 937-4140 Res.

MENDOCINO HEADLANDS STATE PARK IN-FORMATION CEN-TER

The historic Ford House is the Mendocino Headlands State Park Information Center run by Mendo Parks as a museum, gift shop and information center. It is open daily year around from 11am - 4pm. Picnic tables, foot trails and expansive views of the Mendocino Coast make this a popular stop for visitors. Remember to be careful of the cliffs and never turn your back on the ocean because of sleeper waves !! Keep yourself, your pets and loved ones safe , , ,
45035 Main Street, P.O. Box 1387, Mendocino, CA. 95437 Telephone: (707) 937-5397

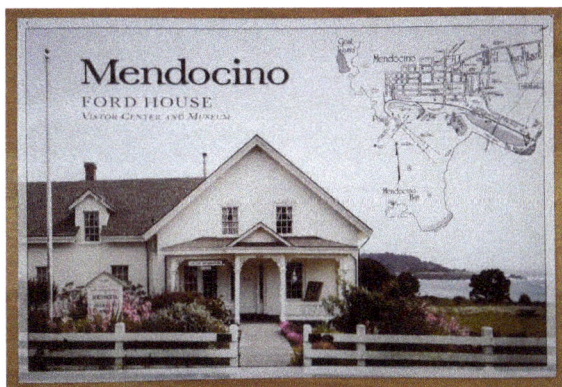

MENDOCINO HOTEL and HILL HOUSE INN

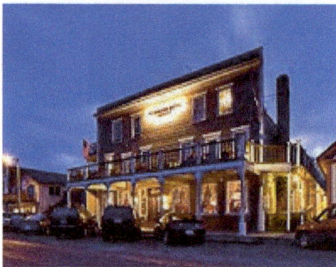

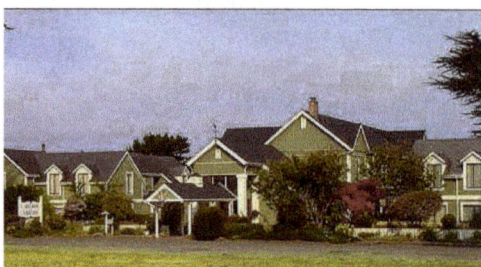

Both the Mendlocino Hotel and Hill House Inn have new owners, are being remodeled and have new names - THE CLIFFSIDE INN and HILLSIDE INN. The historic Mendocino Hotel, which is on Main Street facing Mendocino Bay and Big River offers 26 rooms upstairs ($129 - $309/2 weekdays, $365 weekends) and to the north are three architecturally recreated Garden Cottages with 25 rooms equipped with fireplaces or wood stoves, balconies, and garden views. The historic and spacios waiting room has a large fireplace and comfortable sofas. Many locals have fond memories of dining and drinking at the hotel.

Many of the 44 rooms of Hill House Inn have sweeping views of the Pacific, Mendocino Headlands, meadows and gardens. All rooms have private baths and direct dial telephones. Some rooms have fireplaces. color TV's, king sized beds or 2 full-size beds (room rates for 2 from $100). In the chapel/conference room where weddings and small groups are hosted. Rooms are still available - please check their websites for availability and room rates.

$$-$$$ MENDOCINO HOTEL
Hotel Rooms & Suites   *45080 Main St., Mendocino, CA 95460*
http://www.mendocinohotel.com *(707) 937-0511 / (800) 548-0513 Res. Advised*
$$-$$$ HILL HOUSE INN   *Box 625, 10701 Palette Dr., Mendocino, CA.*
Hotel Rooms & Suites   *44 rooms, ocean views, private phones & TV.*
http://www.hillhouseinn.com/   *(707) 937-0554 Reservation Necessary*

DICK'S PLACE - A Full Bar and Meeting Place for Adventure
$-$$ DICK'S PLACE   *45070 Main St., Mendocino, CA. 95460*
Full Bar, TVs and Pool Tables   *Open daily 11:30am - Midnight, on weekends*
Friday and Saturday night untill 2am   *(707) 937-6010 Information*

FLOW RESTAURANT and LOUNGE
Flow is Mendocino's water tower restaurant with exquisite ocean views. Starters, soups & salads and hand tossed pizzas are served from 3 pm. Early choices are Pacific cod chowder, Caesar salad, roasted beet & arugula salad and fried calamari. Dinner entrees include San Francisco style cioppino, ginger & turmeric chicken thighs, Covelo grass-fed beef burger, fish or prawns and chips, zucchini noodles with roasted butternut squash, and grilled rib eye with wild mushrooms (from $9 - $35). A nice wine list, craft beer and a selection of hard liquor.

$-$$ FLOW CAFE   *4504 Main Street, Mendocino, CA 95460*
California Cuisine with Vegetarian   *Open daily 11am - Closing*
http://www.mendocinoflow.com   *707) 937-3569 Res./ Orders to go.*

MacCALLUM HOUSE RESTAURANT and INN

This elegant victorian is home to the Mac Callum House Inn and Restaurant. You can view the menu and rooms by visiting their website. The "Mac House" is located at at 45020 Albion St., Mendocino, CA. 95460 Restaurant/Lodging (707) 937-0289 Reservations Advised http://www.maccallumhouse.com

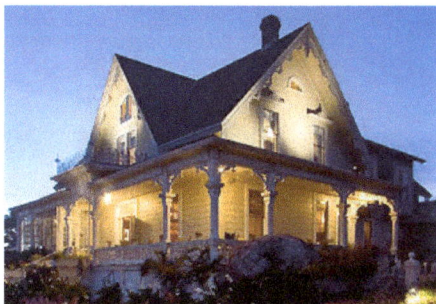

MENDOCINO JEWELRY STUDIO

Mendocino Jewelry Studio features art jewelry that has been hand crafted by local artists whose names are proudly displayed with their unique works. Nancy Gardner, proprietress, received her silver & gold master craftsman status in Lisbon, Portugal prior to moving to the Mendocino coast. For the last 25 years, Nancy has been showing her own exquisite, hand fabricated art jewelry along with fourteen other local art jewelers. Whether you are looking for something new, want to re-imagine something old or custom create your own design, visit Nancy at Mendocino Jewelry Studio on Main Street in the heart of Mendocino.

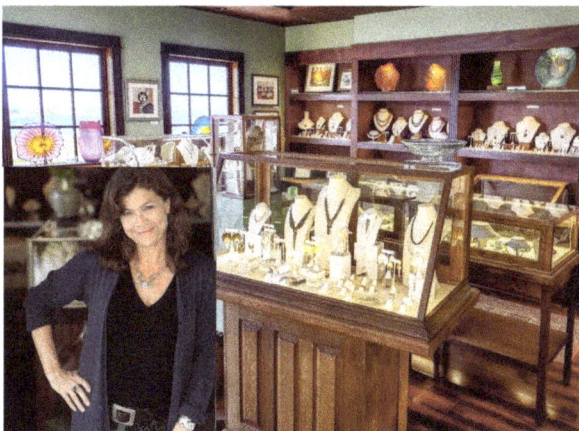

$$ - $$$ MENDOCINO JEWELRY STUDIO

Jewelry & Fine Art in their Oceanview Gallery   *Email:gardner@mcn.org*
45104 Main Street., Mendocino, CA. 95460   *Open Daily from 11am - 5pm*
http://www.mendocinojewelry.com   *(707) 937-0181*

MENDOCINO GEMS JEWELRY

Mendocino Gems Gallery and Studio is a inspirational showroom that features fine handcrafted jewelry by owner Judith Beam and other local precious stone, silver and goldsmiths. A profound display of mixed media jewelry will dazzle your eyes. Lapis, moonstone, saphire, rubies, diamonds, pearls and mineral stones set on gold, silver, tapestry and stone are displayed. Judith is a very knowledgeable gemologist and understands that each person needs different mineral stones at different times in their life; often for healing or rights of passage and for reasons of the heart, mind and spirit.

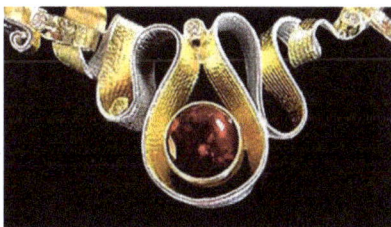

$-$$$ MENDOCINO GEMS GALLERY   *Jewelry and Precious Stones*
10483 Lansing Street, Mendocino, CA 95460   *Seasonal Hours 10:30 - 5:30*
Major Credit Cards and Cash   *judithbeam@gmail.com*
http://www.mendocinogems.com/   *(707) 937-0299 Info and Appointments*

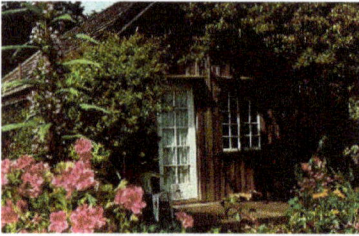

MENDOCINO VILLAGE COTTAGES

Wonderful cottages are situated on the northwest corner of Mendocino, bordering acres of unspoiled coastal headlands. The oceanview "New House" has a wonderful skylight loft, wood stove, rocking chairs, fully equipped kitchen outdoor BBQ area and sundeck with secluded backyard and flower garden; sleeps 4 and rents from $165 for 2 with weekly rates from $950. The spacious "Green House" is great for a small famiy or groups of up to 4 and rents for $185/2 and $1,025 per week. Two bedrooms, fully equipped kitchen, Franklin stove, living room and large oceanview picture window make it your home away from home. The cozy "Garden Studio" is ideal for solo kindred spirits or couples ($85 weekends and $80 mid-week). Your gracious host is artist Gisela Linder.

$$ MENDOCINO VILLAGE COTTAGES

Housekeeping Cottages   P.O. Box 1295, Mendocino, CA.95460
http://www.mendocinovillagecottages.com   (707) 937-0866 Res, Advised

FOG EATER CAFE

"Fog Lites" might be a better name for the Fog Eater Cafe. This upstart cafe is so good that they need to get "some ribbin." Fog Eater offers uncommon dishes that dedicated vegetarians love. Dining is indoors in the tiny dining room or on the back patio. The cafe serves fancy beans & rice, BBQ lima beans, cornbread, creole mac n' cheese, grilled cabbage, fried blue oyster mushrooms with mashed potatoes, fava green gravy and braised greens. Small plates include collard rolls (green garlic & coconut rice with beet cream and pumpkin seeds), soup du jour (spicy tomato carrot with cilantro pesto), spring salad and biscuit sliders ($9 - $25). Happy hour features red and white wines, seasonal beer and the house cocktail. Desserts include banana pudding, strawberry rhubarb pie and chocolate moon pie.

$-$$ FOG EATERS CAFE   45104 Main St., Mendocino, CA. 95460

Vegetarian - Fresh Local Organic Foods, Indoor/Outdoor Dining or To Go
http://www.fogeatercafe.com   (707) 397-1806 Reservations & Orders

MENDOCINO MARKET

Founded by Alvin Mendosa then sold to opera singers and native San Franciscans Matthew and Elaine Miksak, the Mendocino Market today is owned by Sandy Triplet. Her emphasis is on supplying organic, wild, healthy and nitrate free meats, seafood, fruits and vegetables. Wall menu's adjacent the front porch of the big 1870's farm house let you know what the fresh catch of the day and the daily homemade soup or sandwich is. Organic coffee is always on. Choices vary, but may include red snapper, fresh crab (in season), pasta with prawns and scallops, smoked salmon and albacore, country coleslaw, German potato salad and one of the best vegetarian sandwiches on the Mendocino Coast. The market is ideal for food to go, road snacks or picnics for the beach or forest.

$-$$ MENDOCINO MARKET   45051 Ukiah St., Mendocino, 95460

Market, Cafe & Gourmet Delicatessen   Open 11am to 4:30pm - closed Sunday
Credit cards & cash   (707) 937-FISH (3474) Sit Down or To Go

CORNERS of the MOUTH

Corners of the Mouth is a ½ block off Lansing in the historic red church on Ukiah Street. The help is cheerful, informed, and enlightened. This worker's collective is run from the premise of co-operation and consciousness. The staff have your health in mind, with an array of local and organic produce. A large selection of edible and medicinal organic herbs are showcased as well as tinctures and essential oils. There is a personal care section, a full line of bulk grains, herbs, pet food, canned goods, tofu, yogurt, cheese, milk, packaged meat, frozen food, juice, and beverages. A northern California icon, "Corners" has been serving organic and natural foods for over 40 years.

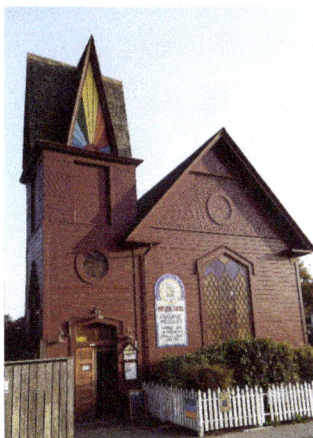

$-$$$ CORNERS of the MOUTH   45015 Ukiah Street, Mendocino, CA 95460
Full Service Health Food Store, Fresh Organic GMO Free Food & Good Cheer
Open daily 8am - 8pm   http://www.corners.com   (707) 937-5345

GARDEN BAKERY

This small, but beautiful setting is a great place to start the day with delicious cinnamon rolls, donuts, bear claws, fruit or plain muffins and scones. The proprietors serve nutritious breakfast burritos, tostadas, pork or beef burritos, with fresh made salsa and hot coffee. The secluded and terraced garden area is a nice place for you and your family or pets to "wake up the morning".

$ GARDEN BAKERY   10450 Lansing St., Mendocino, CA. 95460
Fresh Baked Goods, Mexican Entrees, Coffee   (707) 937-3140

TRILLIUM RESTAURANT and the BLUE HERON INN

Trillium Restaurant is know for exceptional cuisine, highlighting the bounty of organic farms, ranches and fishermen. The wine and craft beer list is very adequate. Lunch includes aperitifs, appetizers, sandwiches such as the Trillium BLT, Caprese toast with prawn & avocado sandwich and local rock cod fish tacos. Dinners include seared albacore tuna, the local cheese plate and grilled asparagus appetizers followed by beet & strawberry salad or the grilled Caesar. Entrees include grilled swordfish, grass fed flat iron steak, crispy skinned wild king salmon, grilled pork chop with fingerling potatoes, with marinade and peach ginger chutney. Delicious desserts are all homemade. Outdoor seating in the garden or deck with views of the ocean, makes dining here very pleasant. Upstairs from the restaurant are three guest rooms, two of which have ocean and garden views. The third room has views of Mendocino Village and its own private bath. Private and share bath rooms rent from $150 per night weekends and $110 - $135 mid week.

$$ BLUE HERON INN and TRILLIUM RESTAURANT
Cafe and Inn   571 Ukiah St., Mendocino, 95460
https://www.trilliummendocino.com/   (707) 937-4323 Reservations

FRANKIES PIZZA and ICE CREAM PARLOR

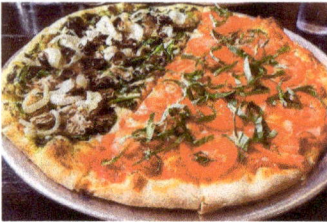

This environmentally conscious, child and dog friendly, fun haven is centrally located in the village of Mendocino. Frankie's offers reasonably priced organic comfort food. This combination café - hang out, features indoor/outdoor seating and is a great place to take a break or plan the rest of your day. Food is also available to go. There's something for everyone at Frankie's; organic coffee and tea, locally made award winning ice creams, delicious whole pizzas or pizza by the slice, gluten-free and vegan pizzas available as well. There are hearty soups, salads, delicious homemade falafel and other light entrees. They also have a nice selection of local wines and beers. Most ingredients are organic and locally sourced. The thin crust pizza is outstanding and named after popular surf spots. The artwork rotates every other month and showcases local talent. Free wifi rounds off this great experience. Visit: *http://www.frankiesmendocino.com/*

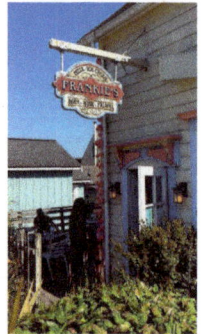

$-$$ FRANKIES   Mendocino Comfort Food, Pizza, Beer / Wine, Smoothies and Ice Cream Parlor   (707) 937-2436 44951 Ukiah Street, Mendocino

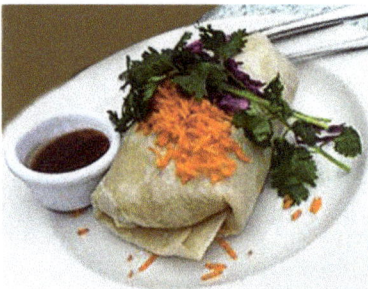

MENDOCINO CAFE

Indoor/outdoor seating with fabulous views of the ocean and forest is an alluring feature of this relaxing, convivial eatery. Luncheon items include a variety of fresh salads, sandwiches, burritos, and soups, with daily seasonal hot plate specials (typically $10-$`20); dinners emphasize fresh seafood, satisfying pasta bowls, and hearty entrees, such as the one half free range chicken baked in BBQ or Thai sauce, served with garlic mashed potatoes and fresh vegetable of the day ($18.95). The legendary Thai burrito ($18), invented by their first chef Maggie Drake, served with choice of tofu, chicken or shrimp is delicious and worth the visit.

$-$$MENDOCINO CAFE   *Corner Lansing & Albion Streets,*
California/International Open daily   *Mendocino, CA. 95460*
https://www.mendocinocafe.com/   *(707) 937-6141 Res. & Orders to go*

HEADLANDS INN

The Headlands Inn, a 3-story New England Victorian "salt-box-by-the-sea", offers ocean, village and garden views extraordinaire. All six rooms (from $119) and the cottage ($250 / 4) have private baths, wood burning fireplaces, featherbeds and lots of nice amenities. The romantic cottage also has cable TV/VCR, microwave, refrigerator and large sunken tub with shower. Next morning enjoy an extended continental breakfast.

$$-$$$ HEADLANDS INN   *Box 132, 10453 Howard Street,*
Oceanview Bed & Breakfast   *Mendocino, CA 95460*
http://www.headlandsinn.com   *1-800-354-4431 Res. Advised*

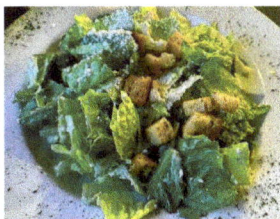

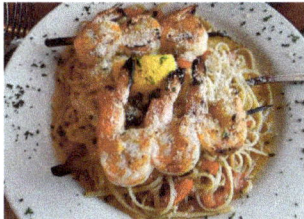

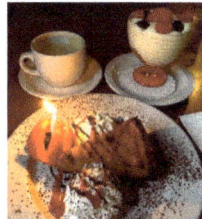

LUNA'S TRATTORIA " Over the Moon Italian Cuisine "

Romance is in the air at Luna's Trattoria. True Italians, Massimo and Marisa, make you feel you are in a romantic villa in Italy's Ravenna, Province. Northern Italian cuisine includes appetizers antipasto misto, bruschetta combo, soups (minestrone and pasta & fagioli), salads (Caesar, smoked salmon salad and insult mist), spaghetti & meatballs, carbonara, all vongole and farfalle California ($16 - $25). Desserts include tiramisu, chocolate cheesecake, cream romagnola, ice cream and custard Italiana with mixed berries. Dining is downstairs by the bar, on the garden deck to the west or upstairs in the romantic opera balcony. The attentive staff promote intimacy and romance so don't hold back. The cuisine is devine, the atmosphere perfect for a very memorable evening under Mendocino's Luna (moon).

$$-$$$ LUNA TRATTORIA   *955 Ukiah, Mendocino, CA 95460*
Northern Italian Cuisine   *Closed Mondays - Call for Hours*
https://www.lunatrattoria.com/   *(707) 962-3093 Res. Highly Recommended*

CAFE BEAUJOLAIS and NICHOLOS HOUSE Bed n Breakfast

Cafe Beaujolais was founded by famous chef Margaret Fox in the 70's. Today's owners, Peter and Melissa Lopez and their son Julian have grown the business by adding an award winning bakery, wood fired pizzeria, farmers market, coffee shop, and opened Nicholos House bed n breakfast next door. Fresh seasonal produce is combined into exciting entrees, gourmet appetizers, soups and salads, but thats not all. Dinners are served Wed - Sun from 5:45 to 8pm, Brickery Pizza 11:30am - 5pm, waiting room coffee and pastries from 7am - noon. Dine indoors or in the garden atrium. Bon Appetite !

$$-$$$ CAFE BEAUJOLAIS   *961 Ukiah Street, Mendocino, CA 95460*
*California - French Cuisine   Also Bed & Breakfast at **NICHOLOS HOUSE***
http://www.cafebeaujolais.com   *(707) 937-5614 Res. Adv.*

BLUE DOOR INN   Six lovely rooms provide accommodations for visitors to Mendocino. Originally built in 1880 as one of the towns most elegant residences, the century old home has been carefully restored with antiques, tapestries, and original art from the less hurried Victorian era. All rooms have private baths and three have fireplaces. The following morning a delicious full breakfast is served. Seasonal rates for are $260 - $300 plus tax. A few blocks away is a sister property, the JD House.

$$-$$$ BLUE DOOR INN
Bed & Breakfast   Box 150, 499 Howard Street, Mendocino, CA. 95460
https://www.bluedoorgroup.com/   (707) 937-4892 Reservations advised.
$$ JOHN DOUGHERTY HOUSE   390 Kasten, Mendocino, CA. 95460
Bed and Breakfast http://www.JDHouse.com   (707) 937-4323 Reservations

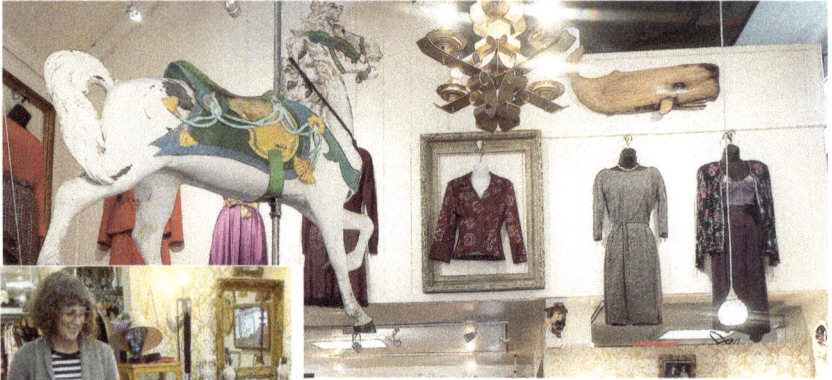

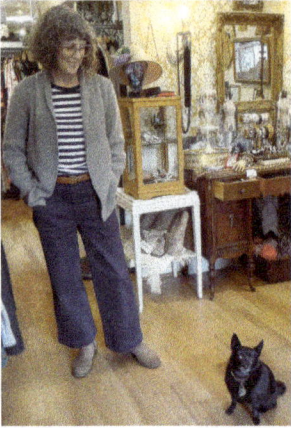

QUEEN BEE MENDOCINO

Queen Bee Mendocino is a uniquely curated vintage clothing consignment store for women and men. Nestled in the heart of historic Mendocino , this small boutique shop overflows with one of a kind pieces of clothing, jewelry, shoes, and other curious artifacts. The real treasure is Melanie Eisemann and her beloved Schipperke, Palie. Customers become friends and purchases become treasures. Contact Melanie at (707) 397-1490.

$-$$$ QUEEN BEE MENDOCINO   *10381 Kasten St., Mendocino 95460*
Clothing and Jewelry   https://www.facebook.com/queenbeemendocino
Open most Fridays - Mondays 12ish-5ish or by appointment.

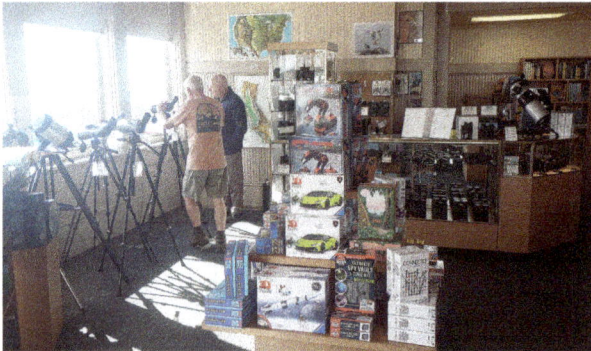

OUT OF
THIS WORLD

For bird watching, whale watching or star gazing, Out of this World has all the right stuff. Enter the showroom with science lab and telescope viewing room. Jump from eye piece to eye piece until you find the perfect spotter or telescope for your needs. Prices are as good (or better) than the internet! Also featured are microscopes and science toys, chemistry labs, circuitry kits, gyroscopes, rockets, and robot building sets; plus a full selection of anatomy books and charts, math games and science books and a unique selection of strategy games and brain-busting puzzles - for all ages.

$-$$$ OUT OF THIS WORLD *Main at Kasten Street, Mendocino, 95460*
Telescopes, Binoculars, Science & Anatomy Kits   Open Daily 10am - 5pm
https://outofthisworldshop.com/   (707) 937-3335 Information & Sales

THE OUTDOOR STORE

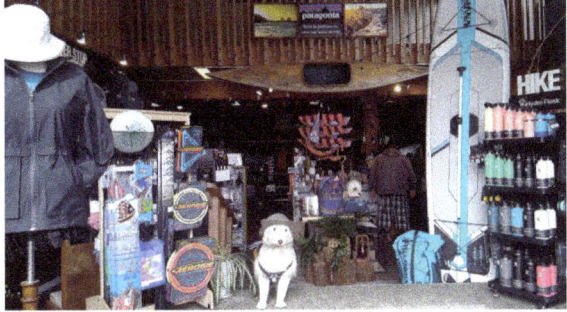

Shop adventure at the Outdoor Store in Fort Bragg and Mendocino where the beginner to the hard core camper can shop. Try on wilderness fashion that makes you look great, and prepares you for all weather - all terrain situations. The inventory at both stores is extensive - hiking shoes, socks, underwear, pants, shirts, jackets, hats and night lights. Back packs include leading brands, sleeping bags waterproof or not are rated to minus 30 degrees, tents, camp stoves, solar powered lights, grills, gourmet freeze dried food and snacks for the middle of no where. Emergency mirrors (signal that helicopter or drone), water filters and powerful solar spotlights compliment maps and books to read around the campfire or under the stars. Wildfire emergency? Don't forget bug-out kits for the kids, and your 2 n 4 legged loved ones.

$-$$$ THE OUTDOOR STORE   *http://www.theoutdoorstoreco.com*
147 E. Laurel St, Fort Bragg, CA. 95437 (707) 397-7171 Both stores open daily
45000 Main St. Mendocino, CA. 95460   (707) 397-1930   from 10am - 6pm

HIGHLIGHT GALLERY

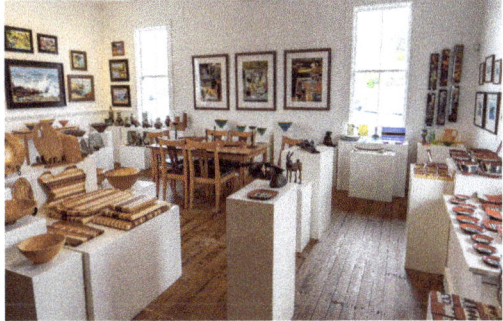

The Highlight Gallery on Kasten Street in Mendocino, has showcased the finest work of Northern California painters, sculptors, fine woodworkers, furniture makers and artisans since 1978. Come and visit them in their new two story gallery on Kasten Street. Everything in the gallery is handmade in America. Highlight also offers fine jewelry, natural ocean sand paintings, turned vessels of wood and alabaster, wire sculpture, art glass and handcrafted gifts. The casual craft lover or serious art collector will enjoy a leisurely stroll through one of California's finest galleries. Perhaps most important in visiting the Highlight Gallery, either in person or at their online showroom, is an opportunity to buy pieces of fine art, hand-made furniture and gifts that last a lifetime. There is truly something for everyone.

*$-$$$ **HIGHLIGHT GALLERY** 10480 Kasten Street, Mendocino, CA 95437*
Mixed Media Specializing in Local Artists   Open Wed - Mon 11am - 4pm
http://www.thehighlightgallery.com   (707) 937-3132 Info.

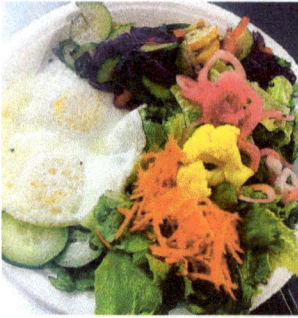

GOOD LIFE CAFE

Proprietress Teddy Winslow learned many of her restauranteur skills from the legendary Lynn Derrick or "Queenie" of Queenie's Roadhouse in Elk. She acquired the former Mendocino Bakery in 2011 and renamed it The Good Life Cafe. Right place, right time is important and indeed the customer waiting line which flows out the front door and down the block proves it. Fresh baked pastries, mochas and lattes, breakfast entrees and a large variety of gourmet meals satisfy your appetite. This a great destinantion for breakfast or lunch and picnic and snack items for exploring the Mendocino Coast.

$-$$ GOOD LIFE CAFE   *Box 1501, Lansing St., Mendocino, CA 95460*
Baked Goods, Pizza, International Foods   Open daily from 7:30 am.
http://www.goodlifecafe.com   (707) 937-0836 Sit down or to Go

PATTERSON'S PUB

Travelers looking for a place where respectable locals and white collar workers hang out will enjoy a visit to Patterson's. Comfort food with a Irish-American slant such as fresh wild salmon, mashed potatoes and gravy, sheppards pie, Caesars, Asian salad (delicious), steaks, homemade chili (delicious), chowder, raw or BBQ'd oysters on the half shell, a dozen beers on draft, premium California wines and mixed drinks are served. Several TVs show sports and news alerting locals to possible ripple effects to Mendocino. Above the long bar hang the mugs of the living and dearly departed. Your proprietors are Mary Ann and Tony Graham Esq.

$-$$ PATTERSON'S PUB   *10485 Lansing St., Mendocino, CA 95460*
Food, Beer, Wine & Mixed Drinks   Open daily 10 am till? (707) 937-4782

$-$$ HARVEST MARKET at MENDOSA'S See Harvest Market - Fort Bragg
Full Service Grocery, Health Food, Bakery, Wine Shop & Local Delivery
Harvest at Mendosa's   *10501 Lansing St., Mendocino 95460*
http://www.harvestmarket.com   (707) 937-5879 Info or Call In Orders

JOSHUA GRINDLE INN

The Joshua Grindle Inn was built by the town banker in 1879 and is set on a two acre estate with views of the Pacific Ocean, Mendocino Bay, and the quaint town. In the main house you will discover a beautiful parlor and five romantic guest rooms all with private baths and deep soaking or jetted tubs, antique furnishings; some with fireplaces. Behind the main house under a swath of Cypress trees and surrounded by lush gardens sits the two spacious and private Cypress Cottage rooms. Both offer large spa baths and romantic gas fireplaces There is also the oceanview Water Tower room. Guests enjoy a full continental breakfast. Summertime hummingbirds visit the flower gardens.

$$-$$$ JOSHUA GRINDLE INN
Bed & Breakfast   P.O. Box 647, 44800 Little Lake Rd., Mendocino, CA 95460
http://www.joshuagrindlemendocino.com   1-844-567-4474 (707) 937-6022

The Gardens of these three inns were lovingly created by father and son landscapers Manuel and Leo Sarmiento. They are at (707) 357-5466.

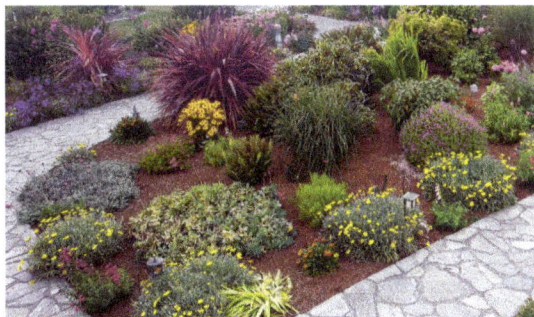

SEA ROCK INN

The owners of the Sea Rock Inn, Susie and Andy Plocher have combined luxury, imagination and down-to-earth practicality to transform this Mendocino Coast destination. The Sea Rock Inn offers 14 cottage units, most with ocean views, fireplaces and whirlpool tubs, neatly set on a rocky knoll among coastal trees and flowers. A few have complete kitchens and all have private baths. Amenities are numerous and include in-room TV - VCR, free wifi, fine books and magazines, snacks, feather beds, natural wood decor and wall to wall carpeting. An expanded continental breakfast consisting of fruit juices, Sea Rock teas, Thanksgiving coffee, fresh fruit, yogurt, muffins, breakfast cakes and bagels is served the following morning. Rates for two are from $269 to $455.

$$-$$$ SEA ROCK INN   *Box 906, 11101 N. Lansing, Mendocino, CA 95460*
Bed & Breakfast, With Oceanview Cottages & Suites
http://www.searock.com   *(707) 937-0926 or 1-800-906-0926*

MENDOCINO SEASIDE COTTAGE & DAY SPA

The Mendocino Seaside Cottage & Day Spa is truly a love nest for intimacy and comfort. Here you can enjoy all the conveniences of a home away from home, but with the awesome Pacific at your front door. Amenities are too numerous to mention, but a few include feather beds piled high with pillows (you can sink out of sight), a sauna - spa, aromatherapy potions, love baskets full of goodies, and some of the rooms are pet friendly. Rates for 2 are from $225 - $761 per night.

$$-$$$ MENDOCINO SEASIDE COTTAGE & DAY SPA
Bed and Breakfast   *1050 Wallace Dr., Mendocino,CA 95460*
http://www.mendoheartcottage.com   *1-800-94-HEART (4-3278)*

AGATE COVE INN

Situated on an ocean bluff, the old farm house appears today much as it did in the 1860s when it was built by Mathias Brinzing. It is surrounded by 10 guest cottages and beautifully landscaped gardens to form a charming tiny Cape Cod-like "village". Most of the cottages feature quaint wall covering, a four poster bed, a fireplace, color TV and a private bath. Each overlooks fresh flowers and the ocean. Mornings the smells of the sumptuous country breakfast, freshly prepared on the antique woodburning stove, combine with the spectacular view of blue breakers giving you the feeling of a once in a lifetime experience. Built at the same time the historic town of Mendocino was founded, the Agate Cove Inn, sets like a gemstone above the sea.

$$-$$$ AGATE COVE INN   *Box 625, 10701 Palette Dr.,*
Ocenview Lodging & Breakfast   *Mendocino, CA. 95460*
http://www.agatecoveinn.com   *(707) 937-0554 Reservations*

MENDO BUNGALOW

High above the Mendocino Coast just east of the town of Mendocino are the 17 Cottages and the two bedroom Big House with its spacious interior and valuted ceilings. Seasonal rates for 2 are from $175 - $450 for cottages and $450 to $800 for the Big House. Accommodations are completely refreshed "Mendo Coast Beachy with a Modern twist". Amenities include private baths some with soaking tubs, queen and premium king beds, large screen cable / satellite TV and firepits for grilling and enjoying complimentary Smores. Mendo Bungalow is family and pet friendly and there is a large grassy knoll to enjoy and sit at the oceanview picnic table.

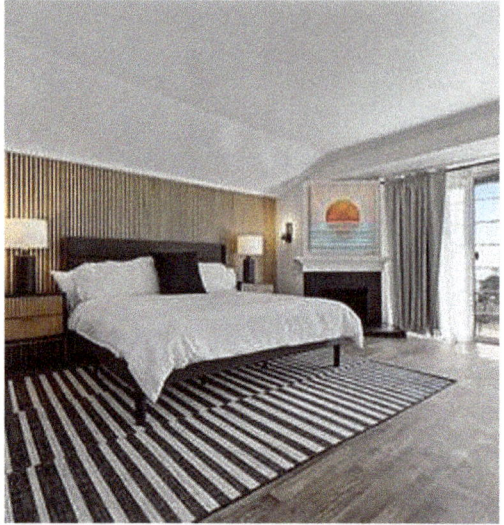

$$-$$$ *MENDO BUNGALOW*

Oceanview Bungalows   *Firepits, King Beds, Oceanviews*
44951 Larkin Road, Mendocino, CA   *Admin@MendoBungalow.com*
https://www.mendobungalow.com/   *707 - 593-0055 Res. Advised*

MENDOCINO WOODLANDS

At the Mendocino Woodlands 3 separate group camping facilities are available to use for activities. Originally created of wood and stone by the W.P.A. and C.C.C. during the Depression of the 1930s, the past decades have weathered the buildings and the combined effect of good design and nature gives the feeling that the facility grew there with the forest. Camp One (usually year-around) is a large spread-out camp with 46 four-bed (bring your own bedding and flashlight) cabins on a hilly terrain. Each cabin is fully enclosed, with stone hearth, closet and balcony. This camp has a 1,800 sq. ft. recreation hall, an "Infirmary" and a "Cooks Cabin"with plumbing & electricity. There are individual and group rates / minimums vary and are often imposed (the camps accommodate 60-200 people). Reasonable rates vary—write for a free brochure or visit the website for the latest.

$$MENDOCINO WOODLANDS

http://www.mendocinowoodlands.org

Box 267, Mendocino, CA 95460
(707) 937-5755 Res. Nec.

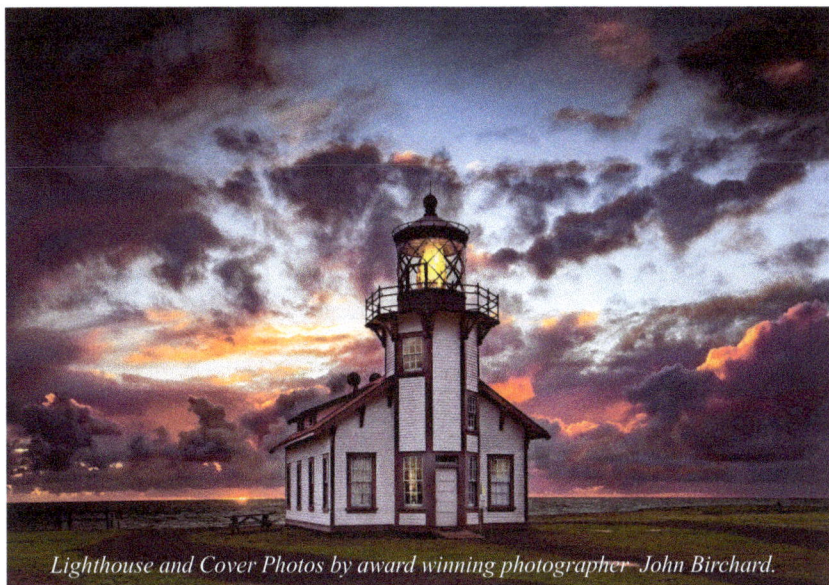

Lighthouse and Cover Photos by award winning photographer John Birchard.
You can see his extensive north coast photo galleries at http://www.birchardphoto.com

POINT CABRILLO LIGHT STATION

Only God knows how many lovers, laying in bed late at night in Mendocino, have looked out their windows into the darkness and stars and been inspired by the flickering beacon of the Point Cabrillo Light Station to the north. Savior of lives, angelic light at dangers ledge, lighthouses around the world have been restored and preserved by well organized groups. This light and fog horn station was originally built in 1909 and restored in 2001 by the Point Cabrillo Lightkeepers Association in coordination with the State Department of Parks and Recreation. The lighthouse, gift shop, lightkeeper's house museum and the marine science exhibit are open every day of the year from 11am - 4pm. The 300 acres of the park and the multiple trails throughout the grounds are open from sunrise until sunset! Soooo . . . don't be disappointed by the 1/2 mile walk through Point Cabrillo Park from the parking lot into potential fog or rain - call to be sure of the hours or check the website. Paths to secret little coves of mirror calm and clear water to stormy seas will reveal mysterious splashes of life in fur and fin in grottos and along rocky crags. Be smart - be safe!

$ POINT CABRILLO LIGHT STATION   *Lighthouse, Gift shop, Lodging*
Historic & Nature Displays   *Mendocino, CA 95460*   *(707) 937-6123*
Box 641, Mendocino, CA 95460   *http://www.pointcabrillo.org*
Pt. Cabrillo Lighthouse Video:https://www.youtube.com/watch?v=GW38ttIeX6c
     Located 5 miles north of Mendocino at 13500 Point Cabrillo Drive,

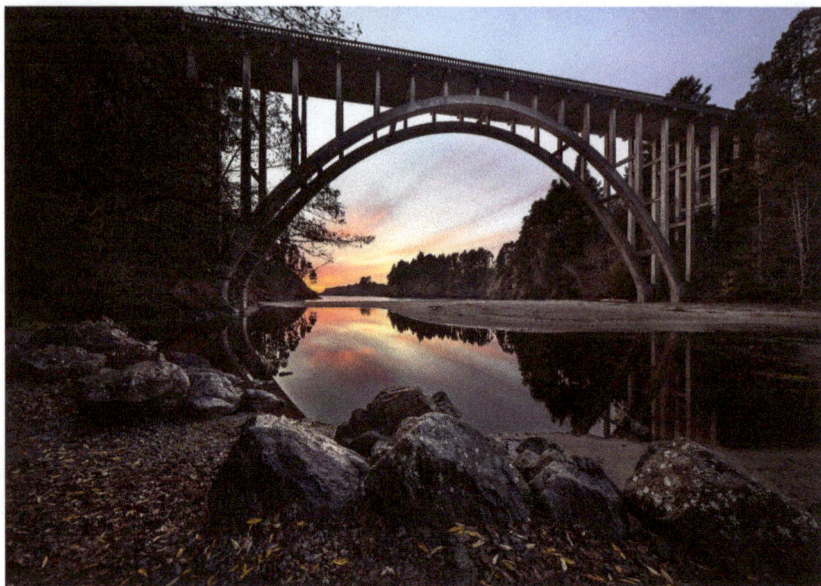

*Photograph by Jeff Trouette of Russian Gulch State Park Bridge "Down Under"
I worked on this angle for a year and then all things finally came together. His work is
exhibited at Prentice Gallery in Mendocino, California. Jeff's photography website may
be viewed at https://jefftrouette.zenfolio.com/*

RUSSIAN GULCH STATE PARK

Russian Gulch State park is located 2 miles north of Mendocino on the west
side of Highway 1. The campground is very small and quiet with 30 family campsites, one which is handicap accessible; a hike and bike camping area; and a 40
person / 10 vehicle group tent camping area. The park is fully developed with hot
showers and flush toilets. Each campsite has a food storage locker, fire ring with
cooking grill and picnic table. The campsites can accommodate tents, trailers up
to 24 feet long; or RV's up to 27 feet long. Rates are $45 / night which includes
one vehicle (additional vehicle $10), day use $8.

There are scenic hiking trails in the park, one which leads to a small but majestic
waterfall, that weaves through coastal forests in moderate terrain. A picnic area is
situated on the headlands portion of the park near a scenic "blow hole" where visitors can enjoy views of the misty ocean spray and magnificent sunsets.

*$ RUSSIAN GULCH STATE PARK   Box 440, Mendocino, CA. 95460
Forest Camping, Hot Showers, Fire Pits, Oceanview, Waterfall, Trails
https://www.parks.ca.gov/?page_id=432   Park Brochure (Link Below)
https://www.parks.ca.gov/pages/432/files/RussianGulchMendoHdldVanDamme-
FinalWebLayout2017.pdf   PARK MAP: https://www.parks.ca.gov/pages/432/
files/russian_gulch_campground.pdf
http://www.reservecalifornia.com   1-800-444-PARK (7275) /(707) 937-5804*

CASPAR COMMUNITY CENTER

The Caspar Community is a model for what a small rural community can accomplish. Well connected financially and politically, the folks who created the Caspar Community Center were compassionate visionaries who combined their wills to create the beginning of a self sufficient community with solar energy, organic gardens, a Tsunami escape plan and wildfire emergency shelter for less prepared refugees. Hallelujah !! The historic school house has a commercial kitchen to cater weddings and special events, a dance hall and stage for meetings and network of creative professionals.

$-$$ CASPAR COMMUNITY CENTER
Events and Community Resources   *Box 17, Caspar, CA 95420*
http://www.casparcommunitycenter.org   *(707) 964-4630 Info*

GOOD BONES KITCHEN

The setting here is reminiscent of a tiny seaside village in Ireland or England where everyday life revolves around the Pub. The owner does his best to recreate that atmosphere with fresh local seafood, choice cuts of beef, pork and chicken; and fruits and vegetables from local farms. Snacks and sides include a toasted bread n butter cheese plate, roasted vegetables, garlic potatoes and uncommon appetizers. Entrees include rock cod stew, roasted chicken, n potatoes, brothy greens & beans and there are delicious desserts. Service can be slow and the moody chef/owner artist changes the menu every week.

The historic redwood long bar used to be the Caspar Inns watering hole for rock n roll bands of the 60's and 70's. A large variety of craft beers, premium California wines by the glass or bottle and all manor of hard liquor drinks are served there. Dining is indoors or weather permitting outdoors adjacent the bar. The restaurant is open Friday - Monday from 5pm - 9pm and there is a "Happy Hour" with drinks and tacos from 4pm - 5pm.

$-$$ GOOD BONES KITCHEN   *14957 Caspar Rd., Caspar, CA 95420*
Oceanview Gourmet Comfort Food with Full Bar & Dance Floor
https://www.goodboneskitchen.com   *Inquire for reservations off website.*

JUGHANDLE CREEK FARM and NATURE CENTER

Jughandle Creek Farm and Nature Center is a 39 acre nature preserve located between Fort Bragg and Mendocino. On the west side of State Highway 1 is the Jughandle State Park day use parking lot with trails leading down to the beach. On the east side are the cozy overnight accommodations of the 1890's historic farmhouse, rustic cabins and camping with kitchen and shower facilities making Jughandle a nice place for individual and group nature retreats. The center can accommodate individuals to groups of up to 60. There are miles of trails along Jughandle creek's watershed, through pygmy forest, giant redwoods, sandy beaches and tide pools. Wildcrafted and domesticated gardens of native plants as well as herbs and vegetables are grown in the nature center. A fully equipped kitchen is available. This is a great introduction for your children to a wild and pristine natural world.

$-$$ JUGHANDLE CREEK FARM & NATURE CENTER
Rooms, Cabins, Camping, Event Center, Ecological Staircase, Nursery, Wildlife
15501 N. Hwy 1, Caspar, CA 95420   *Mail: P.O. Box 17, Caspar, CA 95420*
https://www.jughandlecreekfarm.org/   *(707) 964-4630 Info*

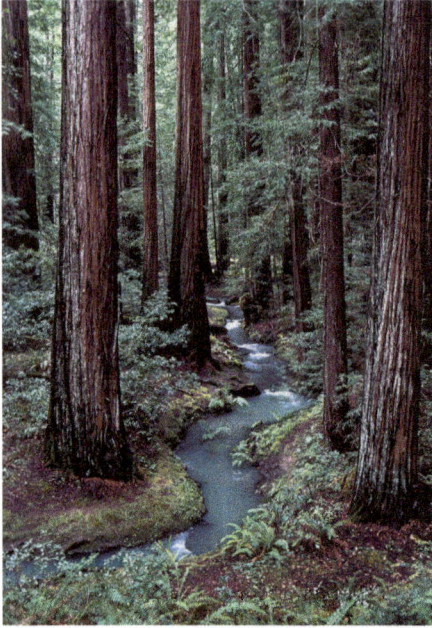

The tallest and the shortest trees in the world grow on the Mendocino Coast. Groves of magnifect redwoods are a wonderful place for deep thinking and problem solving. The stunted Pygmy Forests grow near Jughandle State Park. This photo was taken by Jon Klein. His photos can be viewed at the Mendocino Coast Photographers Galleryhttps://mcpgg.com/

South FORT BRAGG

ROLLIN DOUGH BAKERY and COFFEE HOUSE DRIVE THRU

Located next to the world famous Botanical Gardens is the Rollin Dough Bakery and Drive Thru coffee bar featuring delicious fresh baked pastries, wholesome snack food and every manner of coffee drink. Owners Joanna and John Clemons and friendly staff do a good job satisfying the thirst and appetite of those in a hurry for work or play.

$-$$ ROLLIN DOUGH BAKERY and COFFEE DRIVE THRU
Homemade Baked Goods & Coffee House 18180 S. Hwy 1,   (707) 354-2040
To Go and Baked Goods Sold at Local Markets   Open Daily 6:30 am - 3pm

POMO RV PARK and CAMPGROUND

This campground and RV park is located on 17 forested acres near ocean beaches and numerous town amenities. Pomo offers something for every camper, from large full hook-up sites to a beautiful lush meadow for tent sites. Included in your stay is cable television, mail and message service and WiFi. Propane, firewood, fish cleaning station, dump station, a group meeting room with solarium and coin operated laundry and showers. Pomo Campground "Where the squirrels play and the quail have the right of way." Rates are from $49/RV site.

$-$$$ POMO CAMPGROUND   *17999 Tregoning, Fort Bragg, CA. 95437*
Oceanside Camping, RV Hook-Ups, Store, Firewood, Propane, Security
http://www.pomocampground.com   *(707) 964-3373 Res. Suggested*

MENDOCINO COAST BOTANICAL GARDENS

The Mendocino Coast Botanical Gardens were originally created by Ernest and Betty Schoefer in 1961. The mild maritime climate makes it a garden for all seasons with manicured formal gardens, a dense coastal pine forest, native flora and habitats, fern-covered canyons, camellias, rhododendrons, magnolias, conifers, heaths, heathers, and coastal bluffs. The retail nursery is extremely popular among visitors where unusual and hard to find plants can be purchased. The Gardens is supported by admissions, memberships, plant and gift sales, donations, and dedicated volunteers.

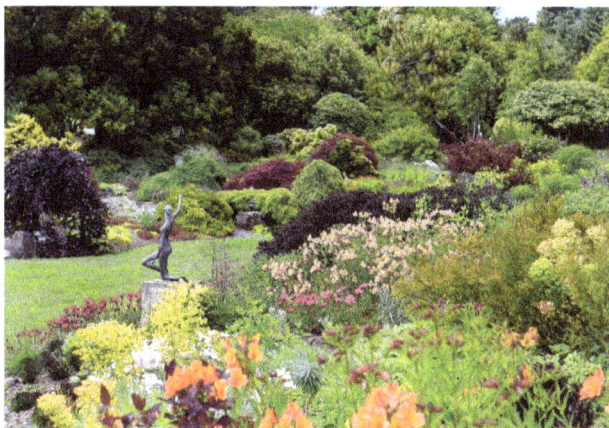

$-$$$ MENDOCINO COAST BOTANICAL GARDENS

Seaside Gardens, Nursery, Giftshop   18220 North Highway 1, Fort Bragg

www.gardenbythesea.org   Open daily   (707) 964-4352

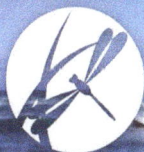

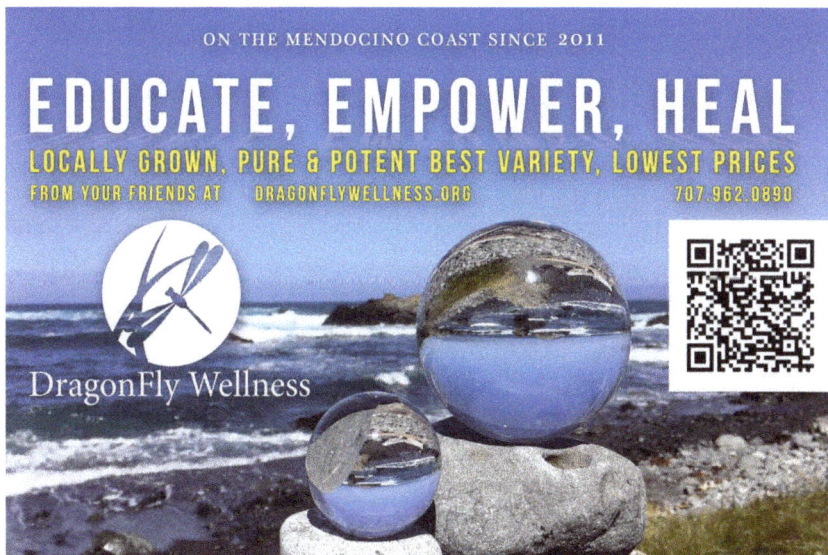

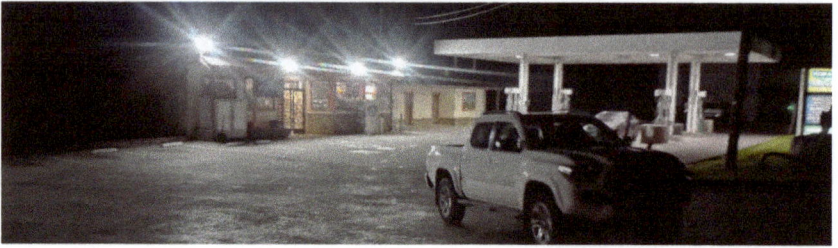

Above is the NorCal Gas Station and Mini Market, which is open 24 hours. Day or night you can get a hot cup of coffee, sandwich, limited supply of groceries and fresh pastries. There is a micro wave to heat food and an ATM Machine. Propane (refills 9am - 7pm) and diesel is available and there is a bathroom. It is well lite at night for security and to illuminate homeless people in dark clothes to prevent them or their dogs from being hit and killed on State Highway 1. Their on-site generator insures you can get gas and supplies during PGE black-outs or wildfire events.

GAS STATIONS, MINI - MARKETS and PROPANE SUPPLIERS
Abbreviations: G- Gasoline P- Propane F- Food EG- Emergency Generator
Albion Store Gas -   Base of Albion Ridge, Albion, (707) 937-5784 GPF, EG
Chevron Station -   810 S. Main, Fort Bragg 95437 (707) 964-5174 GPF, EG
Cleone Store & Gas -   24400 N. Hwy 1, Cleone Store (707) 964-2707   GF
Little River Store Gas -   7746 Hwy 1, Little River, (707) 937-5133 GF
NorCal Gasoline & Mini Market -18770 N. Hwy 1, FB (707) 964-0977 GPF, EG
Open 24 Hours / Hot Food & Coffee / ATM
Noyo Gas & Mini Mart -   1004 Main, Fort Bragg (707) 962-9133 GPF
Red Rhino & Mini Market -   710 S. Main, Fort Bragg (707) 964-5157   GPF
Schlafer's Gas & Repair - Mendocino   Auto Repair (707) 937-5865 G, EG
Speedex Sinclair Gas & Mini Market -   863 N. Main, FB (707) 964-7364 GF
Also Home to Cravin's Indian Food Restaurany by Dennys
Speedway Express & Mini Mart -   18475 N. Hwy 1, FB (707) 964-7051 GPF
Located at the Round-About south of Fort Bragg
Westport Market & Gas - 38921 N. Coast Hwy 1, Westport (707) 964-2872 GF

COAST MOTEL and HEALING CENTER
The owners of the Coast Motel have turned their facility into a destination for lodging and healing. There is more than meets the eye here so expect the unexpected. Amenities include in-room phones, purified water, in-room refrigerator, coffee, private baths, cable color TVs to view self-help tapes and kitchenettes. Please inquire about the special detox and extended stay rates. Across the highway is dog-friendly Hare Creek Beach. Regular travelers will find the motel is a pleasant stay with rates for two from $95. There is even a heated swimming pool and 4 acres of wooded back yard to explore.

$$-$$$ COAST MOTEL & HEALING CENTER   *18661 Highway 1,*
Motel Rooms, Spa & Pool   *Fort Bragg, CA 95437*
http://www.mendocinocoastmotel.com   *(707) 964-2852 Reservations*

HARE CREEK BEACH - A GREAT PLACE TO TAKE YOUR DOG!

IT'S A "LUCKY" DAY

PICTURED is "Lucky" who is off-leash and *FREE* to run the creek and beach at Hare Creek Estero. Hare Creek Beach, located just south of the junction of Highway 20 and State Highway 1, is a great place to take your family for a picnic. It is very popular with surfers and wildlife watchers, with public access from the south shore. Be careful going down the slick wooden stair steps. Best for day use only, as at night homeless people prowl the bushes, mountain lions have taken more than one dog and sleeper waves are unpredictable. Dog friendly accommodations are at Hidden Pines Campground, Pomo Campground and Shoreline Cottages. Be careful crossing the highway. The nearby Mini Market or Harvest Market to the north in the Boatyard Center sell picnic items and dog food. Espresso, mochas and snacks are at the A-Frame Drive - Thru at the south end of Noyo Bridge. Breeeathe! Run Free! Have a "Lucky" day!

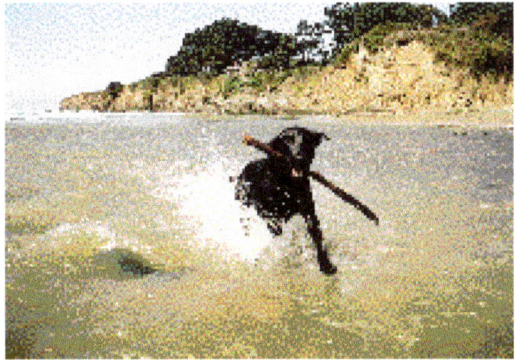

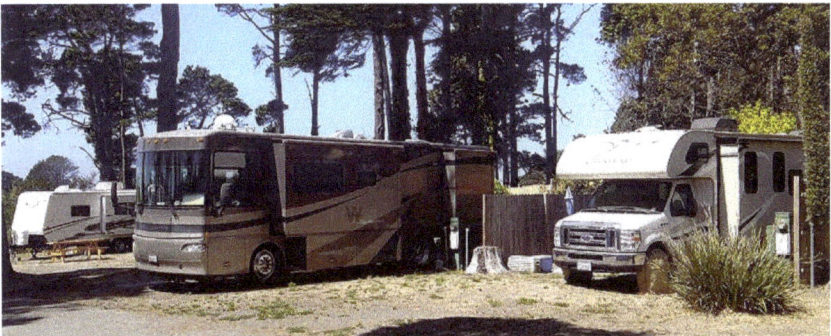

HIDDEN PINES CAMPGROUND and RV PARK

Hidden Pines Full or Partial Service RV Camp Sites can fit any size RV Trailer, Motor Home or RV Van. There are 50 campsites to choose from on a forested hillside close to the ocean for $69 - $99 per night. Campfire Rings, WIFI, Cable TV. Check Ins at the giftshop/lounge or by phone after hours. There is a Movie and Book Library. You will love the quirky - far side website for Hidden Pines Campground. Keep Breathing! And Don't Stop Believing!

HIDDEN PINES RV CAMPGROUND   *18701 N. Hwy 1, Fort Bragg, CA.*
Camping, RV Hook-Ups, Propane, Firewood, Giftshop Store, Hot Showers
http://hiddenpinescampground.blogspot.com/   *(707) 961-5451 Reservations*

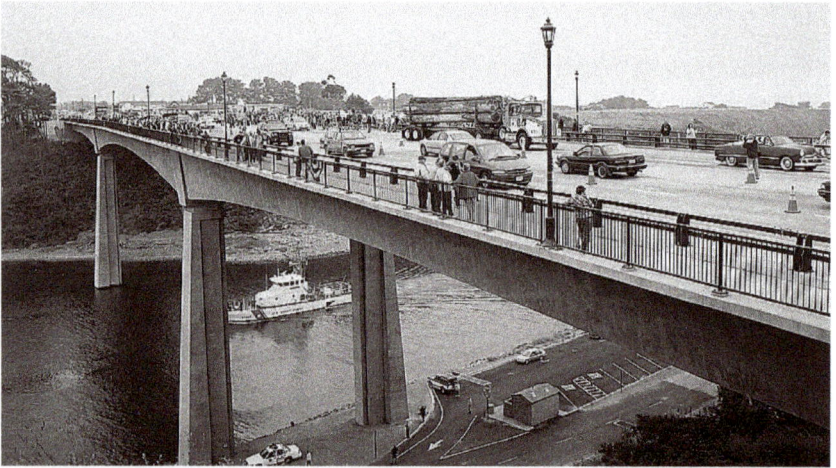

The new Noyo Bridge on opening day August 12, 2005. Everyone turned out and the whole town celebrated. Noyo Harbor, the jetty, bridge and Glass Beach are major attractions to Fort Bragg. You can walk, bicycle or drive across the bridge. Fort Bragg has everything - a river, beaches, creeks, forests and headlands and is America's 1st Bee Friendly City. Numerous restaurants and accommodations await.

FORT BRAGG

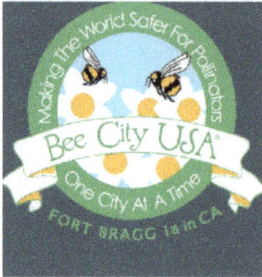

Fort Bragg, located 120 miles north of San Francisco, is a mid-sized city with a "small town personality." The population today is 7,000 plus and growing. It can be reached from the east by State Highway 20 and State Highway 128 and from the north/south by state Highway One. A picturesque wilderness drive is Branscomb Road north of Westport. Rarely does the temperature go over 89 degrees, however days can be windy and winter storms fierce and exciting. Noyo Harbor a premier fishing port. You can charter a boat for fishing or whale watching and kayak the river. U.S. Coast Guard cutter crews are quick and on stand-by.

Visitors can escape the summer heat and stay in a multitude of motels, hotels, bed n breakfast inns, campgrounds, RV parks and vacation rental homes. Lots of places to park your adventure van or RV along the cliffs or in the forests. Keep your vehicle and loved ones (2 n 4 legged) secure during the day and lock up at night.

Fancy to traditional restaurants satisfy appetites from raw-vegan to steaks and seafood. Deli's and sandwich shops abound. Shop for a picnic to go, pizza, sushi, cheeseburgers, chili rellenos, smoked salmon, clam chowder, salsa & chips, organic garden fresh salads, back packer chocolate chip cookies, mochas and lattes; we have it all. Whether looking for economy to extravagant, romantic dinners to casual, you will not be disappointed. Lots of museums, galleries and shops to explore, train rides, world famous "Glass Beach," wildlife watching (people and nature), star watching and beach combing are a few things to do. To the north is the wild Lost Coast. Its no wonder there is a shortage of housing and realestate for sale because everyone wants to live here. The climate, clean cool air and amenities help you relax and settle in. Happy travels !!

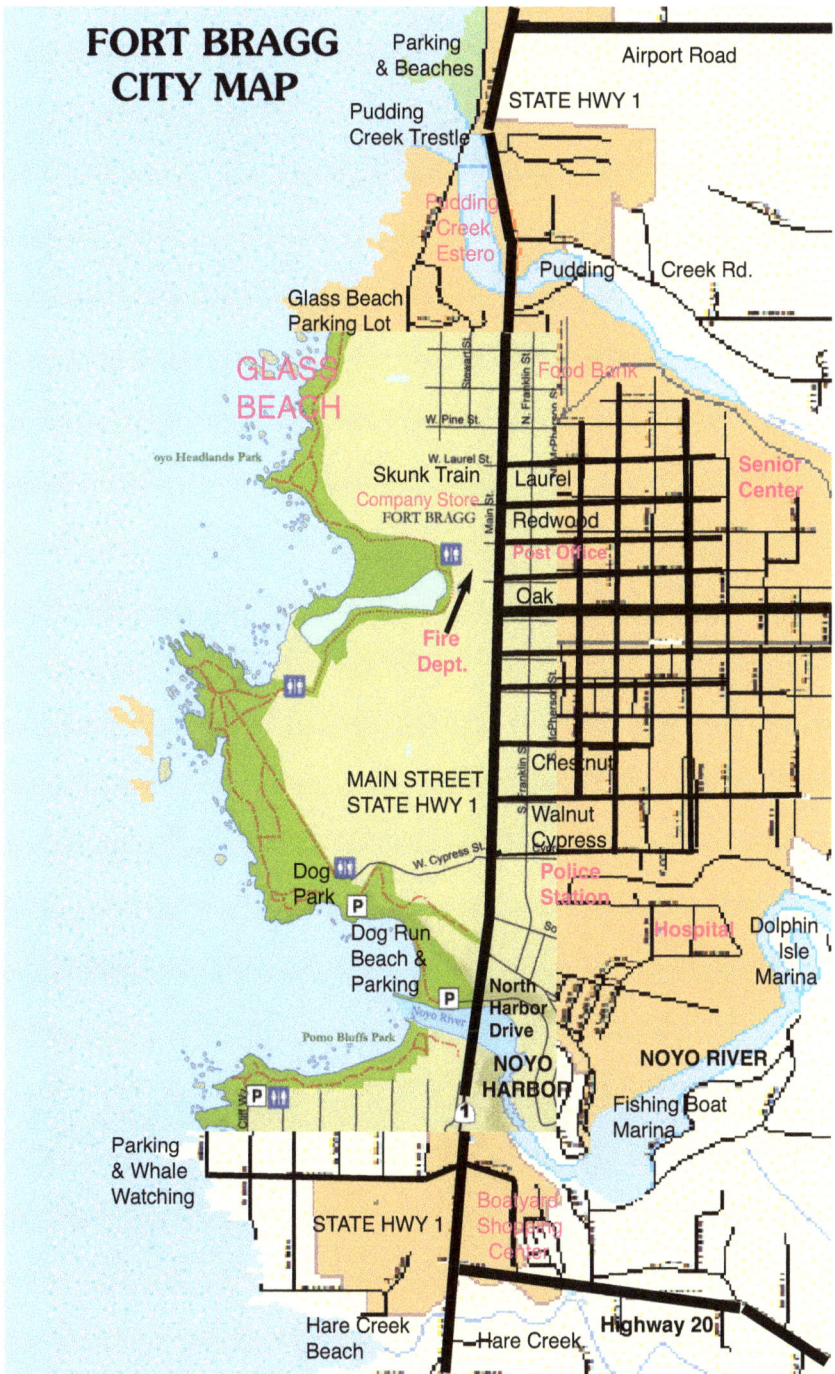

FORT BRAGG CITY MAP

Parking & Beaches

Airport Road

STATE HWY 1

Pudding Creek Trestle

Pudding Creek Estero

Pudding   Creek Rd.

Glass Beach Parking Lot

GLASS BEACH

Food Bank

oyo Headlands Park

W. Pine St.

Stewart St.

N. Franklin St.

Senior Center

W. Laurel St.

Skunk Train Company Store
FORT BRAGG

Laurel

Redwood

Main St.

Post Office

Oak

Fire Dept.

MAIN STREET STATE HWY 1

Chestnut

Walnut

Cypress

W. Cypress St.

Franklin St.

Dog Park

Police Station

Dog Run Beach & Parking

Hospital

Dolphin Isle Marina

North Harbor Drive

NOYO RIVER

Pomo Bluffs Park

Noyo River

NOYO HARBOR

Fishing Boat Marina

Cliff Way

Parking & Whale Watching

STATE HWY 1

Boatyard Shopping Center

Hare Creek Beach

Hare Creek

Highway 20

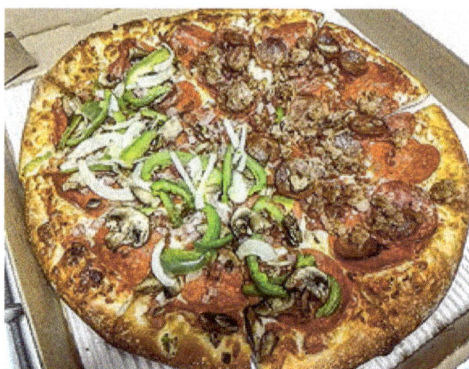

BEAR'S PIZZA and MORE

Vinny's Pizza & More is a locally-owned restaurant located in the Boatyard Shopping Center in Fort Bragg. Vinny's offers dine-in, takeout and delivery. They also take reservations and parties.

Proprietor Eric Poos has a youthful crew that waist no time making, baking and serving delicious homemade pizza's and Italian entrees served with a variety of sauces. Pizza's include the Timberwolf, Carnivore, Vegetarian, Aloha, Chicken & Garlic, Italian Pesto, Cheese and Calzones ($12 - $30). Choices include Mama Bear's Lasagna, Spaghetti w/ Meat Sauce with Mama Bear's Meatballs and Ravioli, 1/2 lb Burgers, seasoned spuds, chicken wings, soups, salads and fresh garlic bread. Premium beer, wine, margaritas, tea, coffee and soft drinks will quench your thirst.

$-$$ BEAR PIZZA and MORE   *111 Boatyard Drive, Suite C, Fort Bragg,*
Pizza & Italian Entrees   *Location: Corner of State Hwy 1 & Hwy 20*
Open Mon-Sat 11am - 9pm, Sunday 12 - 9pm
https://www.vinnyspizzafortbragg.com/
(707) 961-0580 Sit Down or Go
COMING IN 2024
BEAR PIZZA'S NEW LOCATION
Featuring a LARGER ARCADE
and MAMA BEAR'S KITCHEN
111 Boatyard Drive, Suite C, Fort Bragg,
https://www.vinnyspizzafortbragg.com/
(707) 961-0580 Sit Down or Go

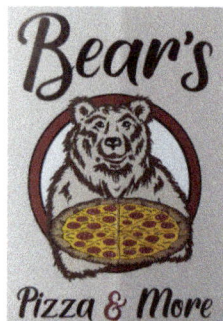

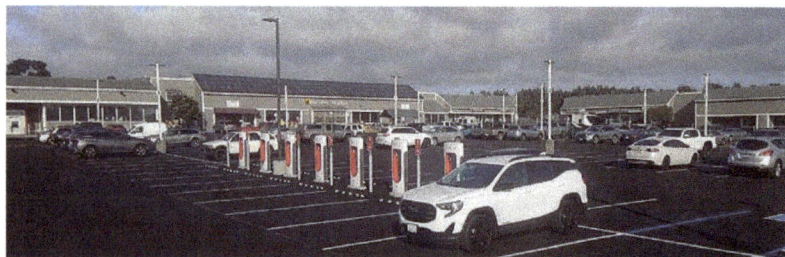

While you are recharging your electric car at the Boatyard Shopping Center, enjoy a pizza and cold drink at Bear's Pizza Parlor and Arcade, breakfast or lunch at David's Restaurant or catch up on some shopping.

FORT BRAGG BOATYARD SHOPPING CENTER
HARVEST MARKET

Located in the Boatyard Shopping Center at the junction of Highway 20 and State Highway 1, just south of the Noyo River Bridge is Harvest Market. Here you can take the word harvest in its literal sense - for a harvest of local grown, organic, vegetarian and gourmet products line the aisles. There is a full service deli serving natural and vegetarian selections, soup, salad, hot food bar, sushi bar, gourmet olive bar, full service meat department and fish market. Harvest has their own bakery, creating fresh baked breads and pastries daily. There are natural supplements, skin and hair care and homeopathy remedies. The Harvest Market catering team includes two full-time florists and a wine connoisseur carrying the most complete local Mendocino County wine selection on the coast.

$-$$ HARVEST MARKET FORT BRAGG / MENDOSA'S IN MENDOCINO
Full Service Grocery, Health Food, Bakery, Wine Shop & Local Delivery
Harvest at the Boatyard Shopping Center   *Corner Highway 20 & Hwy 1*
Deli, Sushi, Natural & Organic Foods   Fort Bragg, 95437
Market (707) 964-7000   Deli: Ext #15 Information or Call In Orders

DAVID'S RESTAURANT

Always packed, you get fast, friendly service from the ladies. Whether huevos ranchos or a traditional breakfast, the portions are hefty. Talkative owner Kira and team have tons of friends and enjoy checking in on all of them. You are greeted by carrots and celery sticks with Ranch dressing to munch while you make your selection. The biscuits and sausage gravy is really good. Combine them with sausage patties, and scrambled eggs and you have a feast. Lunch is more of a soup, salad and sandwich affair with BLTs, cheese burgers, tossed green salads, potato salad, orange juice, coffee and milk. Local artists and photographer's works line the walls for purchase. Davids is conveniently located in the Boatyard Shopping center between Harvest Market and the Thrift Shop. Be careful parking and pulling out as Boatyard Center traffic is not always safe.

$-$$ DAVID'S RESTAURANT   163 Boatyard Drive, Fort Bragg, CA. 95437
Breakfast & Lunch   Open Daily 7am - 3pm (707) 964-1946 To Go

SURF MOTEL

The Surf Motel, just south of Noyo Harbor, offers views of the distant ocean and beautiful flower gardens. There is a cozy lobby for guests to read the morning paper, play games, or chat in front of the large fireplace on wintery days. The clean and spacious units are equipped with color TVs, self dialing phones, in-room coffee or tea, and firm king or queen beds (some with "magic fingers"). The large 2 bedroom suites are equipped with kitchenettes, dining tables and sofa beds. Guests who stay in cozy room 59 can enjoy spectacular Pacific sunsets from bed and then arise the next morning to be greeted by the beautiful flower garden just outside the picture window. Rates for 2 are from $120, with the suites from $180 accommodating up to 6 ($5 for each additional person).

$$-$$$ SURF MOTEL & GARDENS 1220 South Main, Fort Bragg, CA. 95437
Oceanview Motel Rooms & Suites, Gardens   Cash / Credit Cards
http://www.surfmotel.com   (707) 964-5361 Res. Suggested

A FRAME COFFEE HOUSE

Jealous girl friends don't like their men going to the A Frame Coffee House at the south end of Noyo Bridge, The girls that wait on you are easy on the eye as they serve you organic coffee espresso's, mochas or lattes. Its a nice way to start the day. Health food drinks, fresh squeezed juices, warmed up blueberry muffins, croissants, cinnamon rolls, breakfast burritos, sausage and egg sandwiches are also served. The A Frame is for early risers as they start pouring drinks from 5am till 6pm most days of the week. Be sure to tip.

$-$$ A FRAME COFFEE HOUSE   1101 South Main, Fort Bragg, 95437
Drive Thru Espresso, Sandwiches, Baked Goods, Smoothies
Open Daily 6am - 6pm   (707) 964-0199 To Go Only

THE Q - BBQ RESTAURANT

The Q is Fort Bragg's barbecue go-to. Perched at the south end of the Noyo Bridge, the Q's easy highway access makes it great for takeout orders, while the ocean views make a meal at the Q both casual and special. Ribs, chicken, brisket - the Q does all the traditional barbecue favorites, plus locally caught cod, delicate and spicy; in season wild salmon, barbecued oysters, barbecued beef sandwiches and a tasty selection of sides including potato salad and baked beans to write home about.

$-$$ THE Q - BBQ RESTAURANT   418 North Main, Fort Bragg, CA. 95437
California - Mexican BBQ, Ocean ad Harbor Views   Open 11am - 8pm
http://www.theQBBQ.com   (707) 964-9800 Sit down or to go

EMERALD DOLPHIN INN

The Emerald Dolphin offers 43 rooms and suites with king, queen, double queen, fireplaces and jacuzzi spa tubs. The rooms are very nice and offer meadow and distant ocean views. A simple breakfast of pastries, orange juice and coffee is served in the lobby the following morning. Hiking trails, dog run friendly meadows and lofty headlands are to the west. There is also a mini-golf course and meeting room to host groups of up to 20. The Emerald Dolphin sits far enough off the highway to give peaceful sleeps and relaxation, yet close to the Boatyard Shopping Center and a drive thru coffee shop. Rates for two are from $179 - $295. Safety, security and comfort are a top priorities.

$$-$$$ EMERALD DOLPHIN INN 1211 South Main, Fort Bragg, CA. 95437
Motel Rooms & Suites   http://www.emeralddolphin.com   (707) 964-6699 Res.

NORTH CLIFF HOTEL

Located at the northwest corner of the Noyo Bridge with strategic one-of-a-kind views of the river, harbor, bay and open sea are the 39 luxury rooms of the North Cliff Hotel. The grand lobby, friendly staff, vaulted ceilings, in-room fireplaces, spas, custom furnishings and private balcony's make the North Cliff very attractive. Fishing boats and coast guard cutters enter and exit the harbor, weaving like a needle between a series of beacons and buoys which ebb and fall with each seaward swell. The following morning guests can enjoy a in-room continental breakfast of pastries, fruit, cheese and coffee.

$$-$$$ NORTH CLIFF HOTEL   1005 South Main Street, Fort Bragg, CA.
Rooms & Suites with Harbor & Oceanview   Seasonal rates $99 to $225,
http:// www.fortbragg.org   (707) 962-2500 or 866-962-2550 Res. Sug.

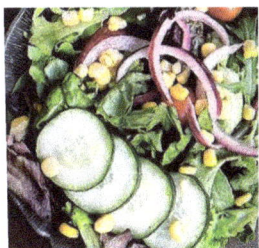

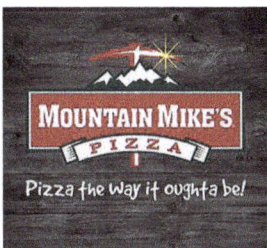

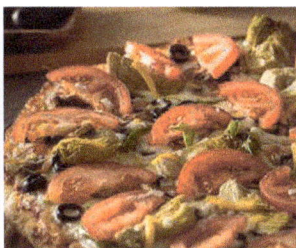

MOUNTAIN MIKES

Tired of fish? Enjoy a delicious pizza, salad and glass of craft beer or wine at the top of Noyo Harbor at Mountain Mikes. The oceanview Fort Bragg Mounain Mikes is a great location to dine at right off State Highway 1 and surrounded by several lodging facilities with economy to luxurious rooms and suites. Guests are assured of a variety of thin or deep crust pizzas loaded with all sorts of the freshest and finest ingredients available; vegetables, fruits and choice cuts of meats (from $10 - $40). Signature pizzas include the Pikes Peak, Mount Everest, Chicken Club, Mount Veggiemore, the McKinley, Diamond Head or just plain cheese. There is also the Cliff Hanger sandwich. garlic cheese bread sticks, fresh garden salads and beer and wine. Servings are generous for later day or late night snacks on your fishing boat, in your RV, or seaside room.

$-$$ MOUNTAIN MIKE'S PIZZA   898 *South Main, Fort Bragg, CA. 95437*
Italian Entrees, Pizza, Beer & Wine   *Open Daily 11am - 9pm*
http://www.mountainmikes.com   *(707) 964-9999 Sit down or to go*

HOMESTYLE CAFE   Homestyle Cafe starts with the ocean views and ends with that satisfied feeling after dining on a really good breakfast. Chef-owner Cordelia Fortier knows how to add those special touches that take a dish from good to unforgettable. Homestyle's famed potato-onion patties, olallieberry pie and everything you could imagine in between is served. Homestyle Cafe - now with indoor-outdoor dining and minutes from Noyo Harbor - is a great way to start a memorable day in Fort Bragg.

$-$$ HOMESTYLE CAFE   790 *South Main, Fort Bragg, CA. 95437*
American Cuisine / Coffee House   *Open daily from 8am - 3pm*
http://www.homestylecafe.com/   *(707) 964-6106 Sit down or to go*

SEABIRD LODGE   The Seabird Lodge offers 65 rooms just one block north of the entrance to bustling Noyo Harbor. Each room has a refrigerator, perk coffee, HBO/ AM FM Radio-TV, direct dial in-room phones, private baths (tub-shower) and game table with comfortable chairs. The suites offer 2 separate bedrooms and 2 separate baths plus complete kitchen. The Parlor Rooms offer 1 bedroom with 2 baths and parlor. Seasonal rates apply - plan on spending $145 - $200 summertime. There are also commercial and group rates for up to 100 compatible people.

$$-$$$ SEABIRD LODGE   191 *South Street, Fort Bragg, CA. 95437*
Motel Rooms & Suites, Buffet Breakfast / Pet Friendly, Travel Info & Packages
 http://www.seabirdlodge.com   *(800) 345-0022 Res. Advised*

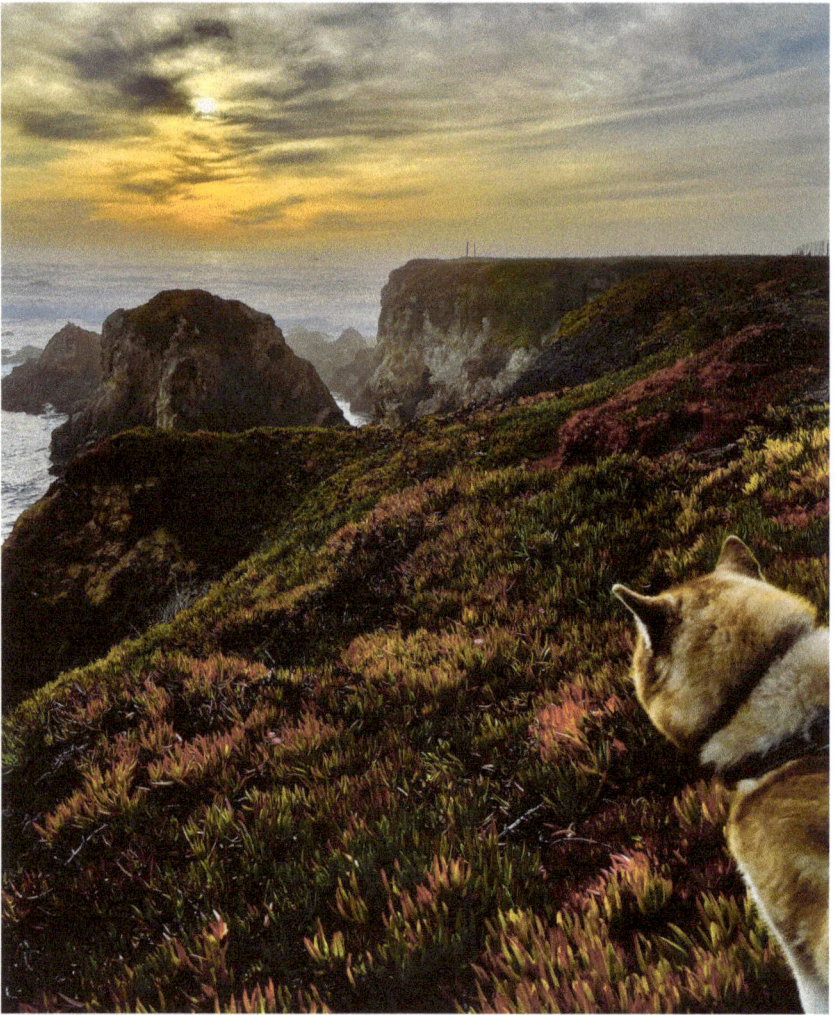

SAYING THANKS TO THOSE WHO HELP US ALONG THE WAY

Mendocino Coast is blessed with a pristine outdoors. Here you can create wonderful memories to share with your loved ones. Many of the owners of the "mom and pop" businesses who serve locals and visitors on the Mendocino Coast are very creative. Rylan Goble, who owns The Shop Auto Repair on State Highway One in Fort Bragg took the above photo of Nakima, his angel dog, on the Noyo Headlands. It is nice to thank the people who help make your vacation meaningful - the chef, the wait person, the motel worker, the car mechanic, the grocery store clerk, etc. Don't forget to say thanks to those who help you along your way. And if you can donate to the non-profits and churches who help shelter and feed the less fortunate among us that are listed in the back of this book.

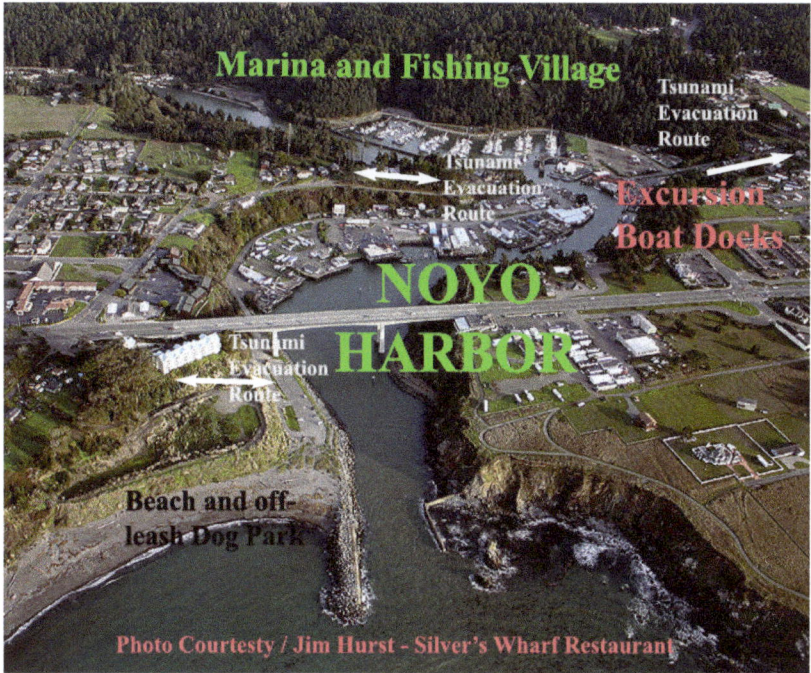

Marina and Fishing Village

Tsunami Evacuation Route

Tsunami Evacuation Route

Excursion Boat Docks

NOYO HARBOR

Tsunami Evacuation Route

Beach and off-leash Dog Park

Photo Courtesty / Jim Hurst - Silver's Wharf Restaurant

SEA PAL COVE RESTAURANT & SCHNAUBELT DISTILLERY

Sea Pal Cove is located in the heart of working Noyo Harbor in Fort Bragg and features outdoor seating overlooking the harbor, where you can watch fishing boats come and go. They are dog-friendly, so go ahead and bring your four-legged friends. Sea Pal is open seven days a week, 11am to 9pm (10pm on the weekends), There is a bonfire every night and a seasonal tent over the dockside outdoor dining area.

They are best known for their Fish & Chips, Prawns & Chips {with wild Jumbo Prawns $20}, Fish Sandwiches, Hamburgers, Cheeseburgers {from $10}, BBQ Bacon Cheeseburgers, BLTs, Grilled Cheese, Clam Chowder {bowl $7}, Chili, Fries, Fried Desserts and have an extensive tap beer list (they have 18 taps).

Within walking distance is Schnaubelt Distillery where crafted spirits are created on site in the old Noyo Ice Company. The tasting Room is open Thur-Sun, 1pm to 7pm. You can set up a private tour and tasting! And yes they are also dog friendly! In the cozy and sheltered interior you can taste hand made batches of Vodka, Gin, light & dark Rum, Candy Cap Mushroom Vodka & Wiskey.

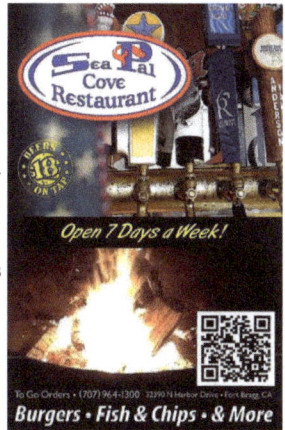

Sea Pal Cove Restaurant

Open 7 Days a Week!

To Go Orders • (707) 964-1300   32390 N Harbor Drive • Fort Bragg, CA

Burgers • Fish & Chips • & More

$-$$$ SEA PAL COVE RESTAURANT
Fish n Chips, Prawns n Chips, Clam
Chowder, Burgers, Beer and Wine
32390 N. Harbor Dr., Fort Bragg
Telephone: (707) 964-1300
https://www.seapalcove.com/

$-$$$ SCHNAUBELT DISTILLERY
Vodka, Gin, light & dark Rum, Candy Cap
Mushroom Vodka & Whiskey.
32425 N Harbor Dr, Fort Bragg
Telephone: (707) 489-4805
https://www.schnaubeltdistillery.com/

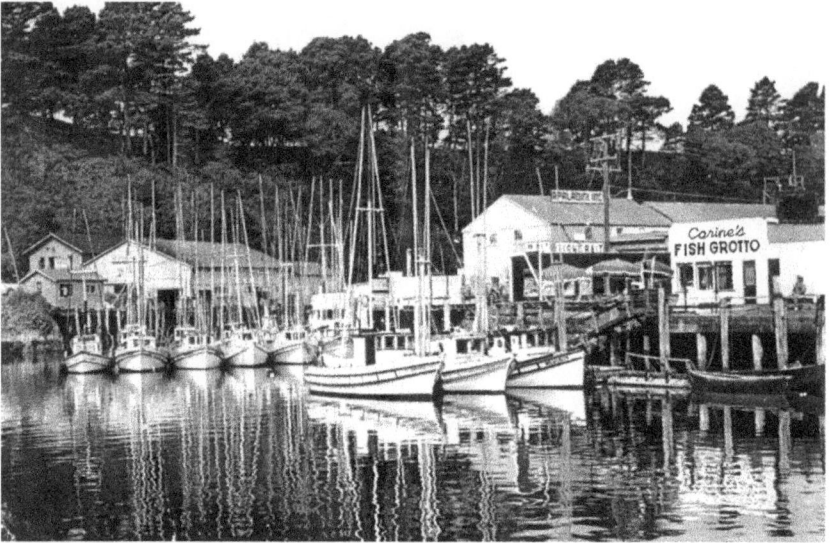

This is a historic photo of the Noyo Harbor Fishing Fleet from the 1950's. Noyo Harbor today is a working harbor and a great place to charter an excursion boat, learn to fish, dine at numerous restaurants, stay at world class hotels or more moderate motels, stay in your van or RV or berth your boat in the marina.

FISHING and WHALE WATCHING on the MENDOCINO COAST

Whale watching season north of San Francisco is usually from December through May. The southbound advanced guard of California Gray Whales including bulls and pregnant cows usually reaches the Mendocino Coast in mid November and December with stragglers as late as March. Cows will give birth in Baja. The northbound advanced guard of California Gray Whales including mothers with newborn calves usually reaches the Mendocino Coast in March and April with slower moving mothers and calves as late as May.

The best vantage points for whale watching are from peninsulas or points that extend well-out into the Pacific from the main continental land mass. Along the Mendocino Coast there are numerous observation points along the cliffs, bluffs and headlands. The Mendocino Headlands, the Noyo River jetty and driftwood scattered north beach offer hours of seaside entertainment as fishing boats come and go, sea lions and sea gulls play in the river's mouth and seasonally migrating whales spout and breach off-shore.

During the annual migrations, whale talks by fishing boat skippers, naturalists and rangers are hosted. Those who want a close up can sign aboard a party or fishing boat at Fort Bragg. Excursions usually cost $50 - $250 per person for adventures just off the Mendocino - Fort Bragg coast or north into the wild and dangerous Lost Coast. Bring cold weather gear, a camera, film, water proof cell phone, and if necessary sea sickness pills. Happy Whale Watching!

BABY GREY WHALE CONTACT!!!

One of the early documented contacts with a baby grey whale occurred with Mendocino artist-divers J.D. Mayhew and Byrd Baker. Their love and efforts were instrumental in helping to save the California Grey Whales from extinction. Byrd and J.D. were men of great courage and passion - we need more such artisan leaders to inspire the connection we have with our telepathic brothers and sisters of the sea. There is a plan to build a $30 million dollar museum on the Noyo Headlands of Fort Bragg to exhibit the huge skeleton of the Blue Whale salvaged from a nearby cove. You can visit the Noyo Center for Marine Science, Fort Bragg's own "aquatic Smithsonian Institute" and discover the mysteries of whales or bring back a souvenir from the world famous Glass Beach Museum. Pictured is J.D.Mayhew making first contact with a baby grey.

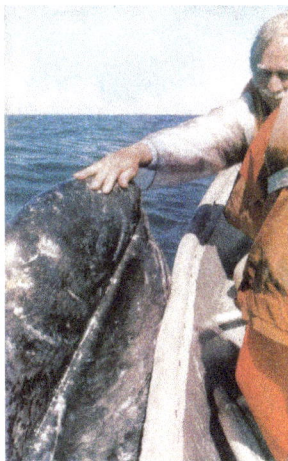

CHARTER BOATS for FISHING, WHALE WATCHING and KAYAK RENTALS
All Are Located in Noyo Harbor on North Harbor Drive or at Dolphin Isle Marina

All Aboard Adventures	http://allaboardadventures.com	**(707) 964-1881**
Ambush 43 Delta	https://www.anchorcharterboats.com/	**(707) 964-4550**
Anchor Charter Boats	http://www.anchorcharterboats.com/	**(707) 964-4550**
Kayak Mendocino	http://www.kayakmendocino.com/	**(707) 813-7117**
(Note Kayak Mendocino is located at Van Damme State Park in Little River)		
Kendall Lynn 6 Pack	http://www.fortbraggfishing.com/	**(707) 964-3000**
Kraken 50 Delta	https://www.anchorcharterboats.com/	**(707) 964-4550**
Liquid Fusion Kayak	https://liquidfusionkayak.com/	**(707) 357-0081**
Noyo Fishing Center	http://www.noyofishingcenter.com/	**(707) 964-3710**
Rumblefish	http://www.fortbraggfishing.com	**(707) 964-3000**
Telstar Charters	http://www.gooceanfishing.com	**(707) 964-8770**

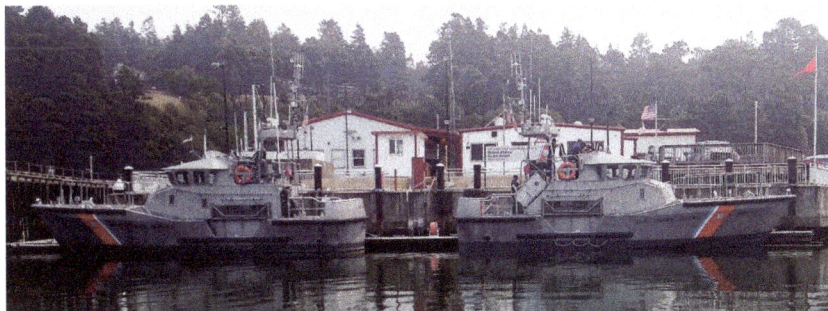

U. S. Coast Guard Rescue Boats: Day or stormy nights they will be there to save lives and rescue those in need. Please support http://www.coastguardfoundation.org

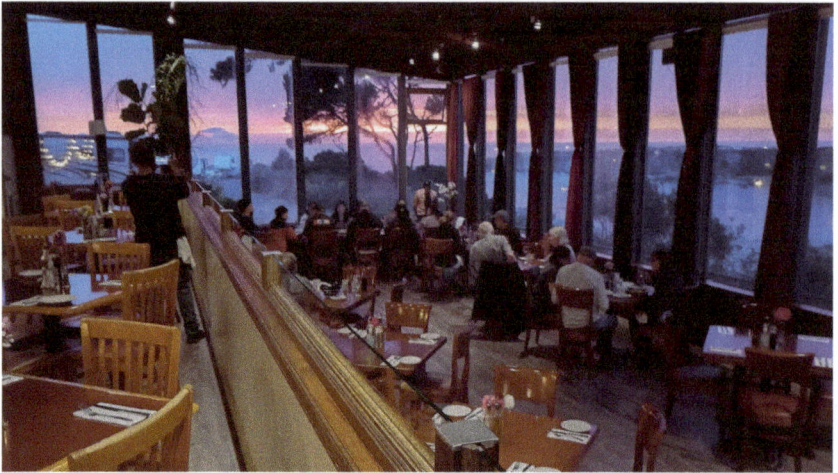

THE NEW NOYO RIVER GRILL

"The best dining room view on the Mendocino Coast"

A dream come true was when the former Cliff House Restaurant opened as the Noyo River Grill. Diners can enjoy the lofty view of the Noyo River flowing into the bay and Pacific Ocean from the spacious glass solarium dining room and upstairs long bar. From "up top" diners are entertained by fishing boats, coast guard cutters, big sea lions swimming in the river below and a sky full of birds. Sunset dinners are especially meaningful and the fierce winter storms only increase your appetite for more.

Chef Guillermo Medina and his brothers Gabriel and Eric focus on healthy foods, having been at Cafe One (a health food restaurant) before

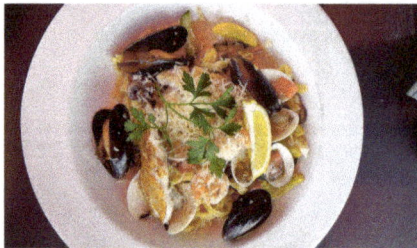

they opened the grill. The menu consists of starters (oysters on the half shell or coconut fried prawns - YUM!), homemade soups or chowder and salads (the cole slaw is devin), homemade tacos (fish, shrimp, chicken or veggie), entrees, wine, beer and dessert (mom's flan, lemon cheesecake or chocolate mousse). I highly recommend the exceptional spinach salad with Mandarin oranges, beets and walnuts with a bowl of their original clam chowder, garlic bread and butter. Entrees include rock cod picacata, Noyo rib eye steak, the Noyo burger and NRG Cioppino (from $14 - $35).

$-$$ *NOYO RIVER GRILL*   *1011 S Main Street, Fort Bragg, CA.*
Mexican-American Seafood   *Sit Down or To Go*
https://www.noyorivergrill.com/   *(707) 962-9050 Reservations*

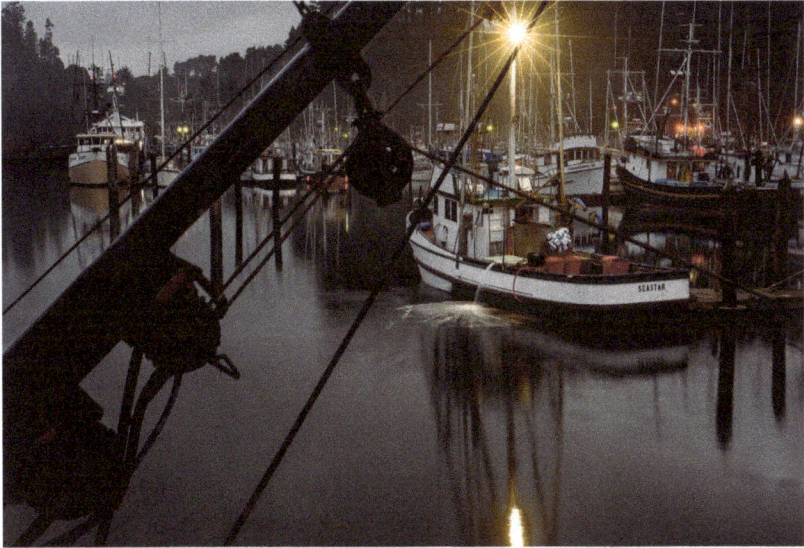

"Good Morning Noyo" is a early morning photo of the Noyo Fishing Fleet.

Noyo Harbor is a working harbor and home to around 180 commercial fishing boats and sport pleasure craft. It is a vital part of the Fort Bragg economy with multiple restaurants, giftshops and lodging facilities. Each year thousands of visitors marvel at the scenery, dockside activity and fresh seafood. Noyo beach is a off-leash dog park and party boats take people whale watching and fishing. The above photo is by Ken Van Der Wende, who is a member of the Mendocino Coast Photo-graphy Gallery. The gallery website is at https://www.mcpgg.com/ or call (707) 964-4706.

PRINCESS SEAFOOD MARKET and RESTAURANT

The Princess is owned by dynamic chef/fisher women who have carved out a very successful seafood restaurant and market. Their fishing boat, the Princess, provides fresh caught salmon, sable fish and in season crab. Ling cod, petrale and Dover sole are purchased from other fishermen. What makes the Princess so good is that its comfort seafood done right. Grilled or BBQ, wild salmon, rock cod sandwiches, fish tacos, lobster

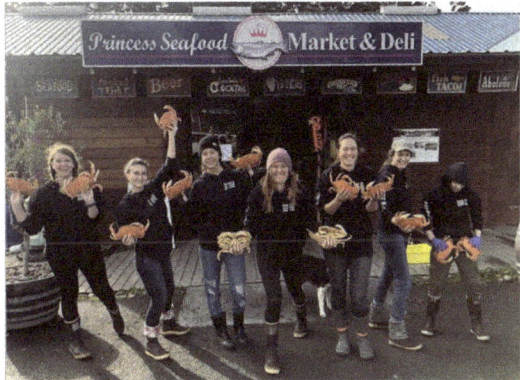

and crab bisque, fresh organic garden salads, cole slaw and angus burgers are served. There are craft beers, premium wine and locally made Kombucha. The seafood market showcases fresh locally caught food. The restaurant is just to the north.

$-$$ PRINCESS SEAFOOD Market   *32140 N. Harbor Dr., Fort Bragg, CA*
Fresh Seafood, BBQ Oysters   *http://www.fvprincess.com*   *(707) 962-3123*
$-$$ PRINCESS SEAFOOD Restaurant 32096 N. Harbor Dr., (707) 962-3046

NOYO HARBOR INN, RESTAURANT and BISTRO BAR

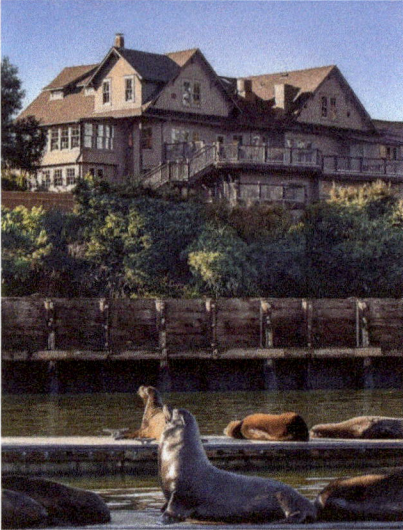

This lofty hillside setting has always been a strategic point to observe the ebb and flow of the wild Noyo River. At the luxurious Noyo Harbor Inn you can enjoy a superb meal or drink while enjoying scenic views of the Noyo River, fishing fleet and abundant wildlife. Luxurious rooms and suites with king beds and lofty harborviews are available all week. The bistro bar and restaurant is open Wednesday thru Monday from 9am - 10pm.

Brunch includes eggs benedict Florentine, baked polenta cake, rock cod sandwich or grilled chicken BLT, flash fried brussel sprouts, soup of the day with house or Caesar salad and the captains's seafood platter.

Dinner starters include wild mushroom ravioli or steamed clams and mussels with wine and cream, Main courses feature stuffed petrale sole with crab, mushrooms and leeks, rack of lamb, surf & turf lobster and filet with garlic mashed potatoes and local vegetables, gnocchi alfredo and the Harbor burger.

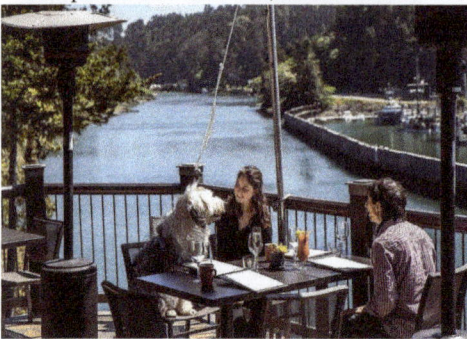

A full bistro bar is quite the show with a large variety of white, red and sparkling wines, plus gin, vodka, brandy, aperitif/digestif, tequila & mezcal, rum, liqueurs, American and Scotch whisky, beer, ciders and non alcoholic drinks. Coffees, lattes, mochas, sparkling waters, teas and mocktails are also served .

The Noyo Harbor Inn can host your wedding, private party, outdoor event with drinks, appetizers and a full menu, or indoor private dining for up to 20 guests. Their experienced team will make your event truly memorable.

$$-$$$ NOYO HARBOR INN
Bed and Breakast, Bistro Bar and
Restaurant, Harbor Views
500 Casa Del Noyo Dr.,
Fort Bragg, CA 95437
Restaurant Open Wed - Mon 9am - Closing
Luxurious Rooms, Suites with King Beds
https://www.noyoharborinn.com/
{707} 961-8000 Reservations Suggested

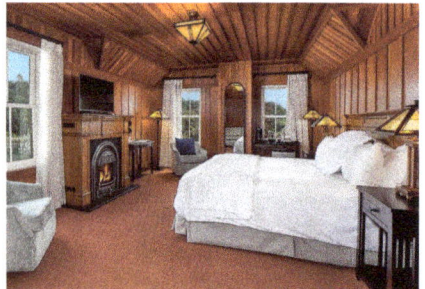

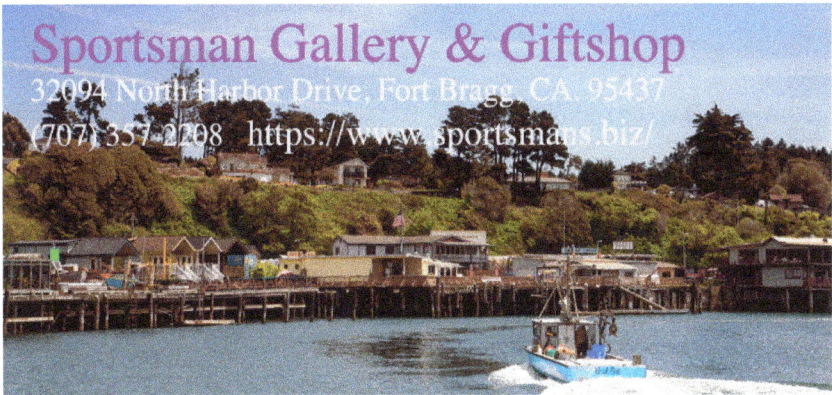

Sportsman Gallery & Giftshop
32094 North Harbor Drive, Fort Bragg, CA. 95437
(707) 357-2208 https://www.sportsmans.biz/

$$-$$$ *PACIFIC BLUE VACATION HOMES & SPORTSMANS RV PARK*
32094 N. Hwy 1, Fort Bragg, CA. 95437 *In Noyo Harbor Near Restaurants,*
beach and dog friendly parks. *Nautical Giftshop on Premises*
Tiny Houses, Vacation Homes, RV Hook-Ups, *(707) 357-2208 Res.*

CASA DEL SOL
Seafood is the heart and soul of Casa del Sol. Located in the heart of Noyo Harbor, Casa del Sol serves fresh, local caught salmon, cod, tuna and crab in season, and delicious, generous portions year round, from straight up fish and chips to cajun fish and steak tacos, as well as many dishes featuring classic Latin flavors and styles. Casa del Sol offers specials throughout the week and is run by a classy crew of restauranteurs who understand hospitality and fine food.
$$-$$$ CASA DEL SOL *32351 N. Harbor Dr., Fort Bragg, CA. 95437*
Fresh Seafood & Latin Cuisine *(707) 409-5095 Sit Down or Go*

DOLPHIN ISLE MARINA
One of the best kept secrets in Fort Bragg lies hidden in a river valley rain forest teaming with birds, seals, fish and wildlife. This secluded RV park and fishing resort is 2 miles up Noyo River with access to the Pacific. Guests feel welcomed to a complete range of amenities including 125 bay and river moorings, laundry facilities, recreation room, cable TV, ice station, paved roads and marine store with coolers full of local beer and wine as well as sodas, mineral water, chilled fruit juices and tea. Hot and cold showers for the gentlemen and ladies are in the campground. Prices are more than fair. The marina also offers gasoline and diesel sales and complete gas and diesel engine repairs. The setting is cradled in the river valley with timbered forests reaching to the waters edge and teaming with the eyes of birds and wildlife watching the human drama below them.
$$-$$$ DOLPHIN ISLE MARINA *32299 Basin Street, Fort Bragg, CA.*
RV Hook Ups, Camping, Hot Showers, Store, Kayaking, Bird Watching
http://wwwdolphinislemarina.com *(707) 964-4113 Res. Advised*

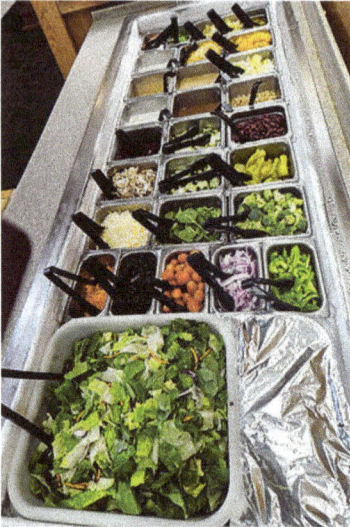

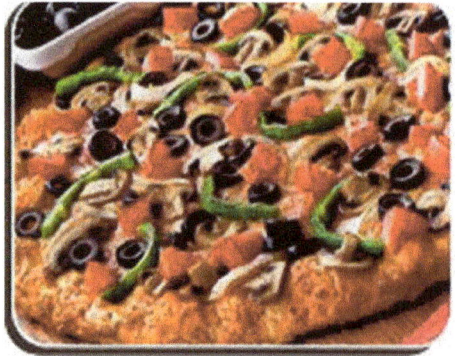

ROUND TABLE PIZZA

At the Round Table Pizza in Fort Bragg, Laud Parks and her committed staff serve up great tasting pizzas that customers crave. They roll their own dough from scratch, add a fresh blend of real three cheeses, and lavishly top their pizzas with only premium meats and garden fresh vegetables on an array of traditional and unique specialty pizzas. By serving a superb pizza and nurturing family connections in a comfortable place to gather, we can all be a part of bringing family and friends closer together at Round Table Pizza.

$-$$ ROUND TABLE PIZZA   *740 South Main, Fort Bragg, CA.95437*
Pizza, Italian Entrees, Soup-Salad Bar, Beer & Wine   *Open Daily 11am-9pm;*
Fri & Sat till 9:30pm   *https://www.roundtsblepizza.com/rtp/*
Sit Down, Orders To Go, Parties & TV Lounge, Order on line   *(707) 964-4987*

MOTEL 6 and ANGELINA'S RESTAURANT and CANTINA

At Motel 6 Fort Bragg you get the works; private room with king or queen bed (1 or 2), wide screen cable TV, stand-up bathroom shower, refrigerator, lots of counter space, heater / air conditioner, indoor heated pool with jacuzzi jetted tub, and an on-site California-Mexican restaurant with cantina full bar, wide screen TVs and occasional live entertainment. Angelina's chili rellenos are delicious with choice of refried or black beans, rice, tortillas and homemade salsa and chips. Other entrees include steak, chicken, fresh fish, potatoes and gravy with gourmet salad mix. Breakfast and lunch is also served. Motel 6 management is big of heart, but run a tight ship. Be safe and lock your car and keep your "Angel dog" on a leash. Winter rates from $65/2, summer $149/2 + tax.

$-$$ MOTEL 6   *191 South Main, Fort Bragg, CA. 95437*
Motel Rooms & Suites   *(707) 964-4761 Res. Advised*
$-$$ ANGELINA'S BAR & GRILL   *400 South Main, Fort Bragg, CA. 95437*
California - Mexican Cuisine, Full Bar, Live Entertainment, Karioke & More
http://www.angelinasmexican.com   *(707) 964-1700 Sit down or to go*

LA PLAYA RESTAURANT and CANTINA FULL BAR

Bright, spacious and lively, La Playa is a great choice for family Mexican dining in Fort Bragg. Or sit at the friendly bar, where a game is always on and the margaritas (now available to go) are always fresh. Diners of all ages are sure to find something to delight them on La Playa's large, traditional menu. A table with a great sunset view rounds out the meal at La Playa, located right on Highway 1 a few blocks past the Noyo Bridge.

$-$$$ LA PLAYA MEXICAN CUISINE   *760 South Main,*
California - Mexican Cuisine / Full Bar   *Fort Bragg, CA. 95437*
http://www.laplayafortbragg.com   *(707) 964-4074 Sit down or to go*

SAFEWAY GROCERY STORE - OPEN 24 HOURS and STARBUCKS

Safeway is a God send for those who need to shop in the middle of the night for something to eat or drink. Besides a full line of groceries and fresh produce 24 hours a day, there are tioletries, cosmetics, soaps, shampoos, first aid, snacks galore, magazines, rental movies and an ATM. Late at night look for the stocking clerk to check out. They also let people safely park their cars and RVs late at night with prior permission.
The next morning **STARBUCKS**, located right next door opens at 5:30am to 6:00am.

$-$$$ SAFEWAY   *660 S. Main Street, Fort Bragg, CA. 95437*
https://local.safeway.com/safeway/ca/fort-bragg/660-s-main-st/grocery-deliv-
ery-pickup.html   *(707) 964-4079 Orders and Information*
$-$$ STARBUCKS   *576 S. Main Street, Fort Bragg, CA. 95437*
Coffee, Mochas, Espresso and Hot Food   *(707) 964-4256 Info & Orders*

D 'AURELIOS ITALIAN RISTORANTE and PIZZA PARLOR

Dinner begins with D Aurelios famous Italian bread, which is baked fresh daily. Pasta meals with very generous portions range from $12 - $15 for a 1/2 order or $17 - $20 full order; with choice of marinera, pesto or alfredo sauce. Meatballs, Italian sausages, chicken and even shrimp pasta are some of the many meals. Options for vegetarians include primavera (fresh steamed vegetables), or pesto pasta. The Pizza ovens are a beehive of activity with over 24 toppings to choose from. There are micro brewed beers, California wines, mineral water, soft drinks and draft beer by the glass or pitcher.

$-$$ D'AURELO'S   *438 South Franklin, Fort Bragg, CA. 95437*
Homemade Italian Entrees & Pizza   *(707) 964-4227 Sit down or to go*

DOWN HOME FOODS

Located one block east of State Highway 1 near the corner of Redwood Avenue and on South Franklin is Fort Bragg's original natural food store. Thanks to founder Stan Miklose, the store will enrich your life with health promoting natural foods, vitamins, supplements, cosmetics and child safe household products. A natural line of medicines and pet care products are also stocked. Much of the fresh seasonal produce is grown in Mendocino County. Delicious and nutritious fresh squeezed fruit & vegetable juices are created right before your eyes. Down Home Foods is open daily but Sunday from 9:15 am to 5:30 pm Mon-Fri, 10 am - 5 pm Sat. A toast to your health.

$-$$ DOWN HOME FOODS   *115 South Franklin, Fort Bragg, CA. 95437*
Natural Foods Store   *Approved Checks, MC & Visa*   *(707) 964-4661*

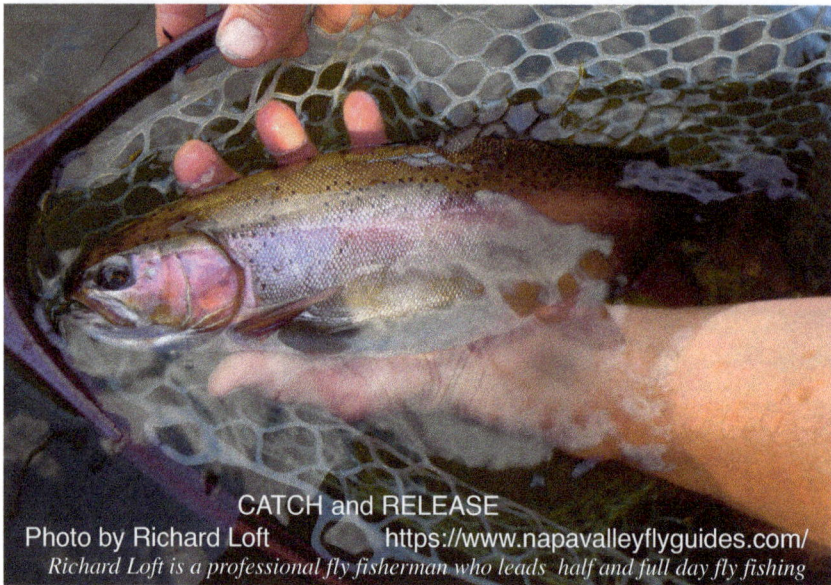

CATCH and RELEASE
Photo by Richard Loft   https://www.napavalleyflyguides.com/
Richard Loft is a professional fly fisherman who leads half and full day fly fishing trips. Contact him at (707) 294-4738 or at napavalleyflyguides@gmail.com

FISH FRIENDLY WINES ARE CREATED BY MENDOCINO WINERIES THAT GROW GRAPES ORGANICALLY and BIODYNAMICALLY

Conscious consumers seek out wines that are environmentally and fish friendly, whereby no Round-Up, GMOs, or petrochemical based herbicides and pesticides are used in the vineyards or wine production. Salmon and steelhead fish that live in the creeks near these vineyards are safe from poisoning. Field workers do not get health disorders from exposure to contaminated air, soil or irrigation water. The following wineries use grapes grown by CCOF organic or Biodynamic standards to make their great tasting and award winning wines. Area Code (707)

1.Barra of Mendocino   https://www.barraofmendocino.com/   485-0322
2.Bonterra Winery   https://www.bonterra.com/   800-826-5092
3. Campovida Estate Winery https://www.campovida.com/   744-8797
4. Fog Bottle Shop   https://fogeatercafe.com/fogbottleshop   397-1806
5. Frey Winery   https://www.freywine.com   485-5177
1. Girasole Vineyards   https://www.barraofmendocino.com/   485-0322
6. Handley Cellars   https://handleycellars.com/winery/   895-3876
7. Le Vin Winery   https://www.levinvineyards.com   894-2304
8. McFadden Winery   https://www.mcfaddenfarm.com/   800-544-8230
   Hopland Tasting Room   13275 S. Hwy 101, #5, Hopland, 707-744-8463
9. Mendocino Wine Co.   https://mendocinowineco.com/   800-362-9463
10 Pacific Star Winery   https://www.pacificstarwinery.com/   964-1155
12 Saracina Winery   https://www.saracina.com/   670-0199
7. Seawolf Winery   https://seawolfwines.com/   494-0312
13 SIP Wine Shop   *142 Laurel Street, Fort Bragg, CA 95437*   472-7092
14 Terra Savia Winery   https://www.terrasavia.com/   744-1114
15 Yorkville Cellars   https://www.yorkvillecellars.com/   894-9177

The Tour of a Lifetime

Finally a luxurious tour of Mendocino County Winerys that create award winning wines made from organic or biodynamically grown grapes. Travel into this rich natural environment from the historic coastal town of Mendocino, past majestic groves of century old redwoods and into the heart of the organic wine country. Tours are one to two days and begin in Mendocino with stops in the Alexander Valley, Hopland, Ukiah and the Redwood Valley. The map below corresponds with the numbered wineries on the previous page. Enjoy the ride and treasure the wine and memories.

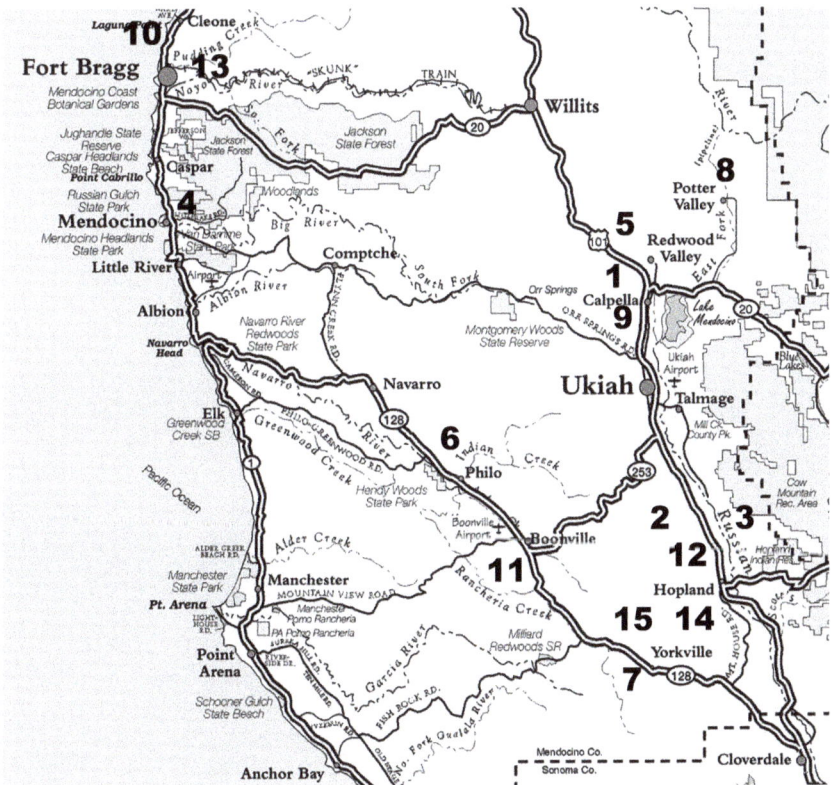

LOST COAST FOUND

Fort Bragg is blessed with many small mom n pop gift shops, bookstores and galleries. Lost Coast Found is all three. Megan Caron is founder and proprietor of Lost Coast Found, a vintage and found object curiosity shop that offers an abundant inventory of vintage housewares along with a carefully curated collection of books, California and studio pottery, art glass and small furniture. Adjacent her showroom is the **Larry Spring Museum of Common Sense.** Larry was a wonderful "think out of the box scientist" and philantropist whose donations helped create the current Fort Bragg Senior Center. Megan feels that "like other former industrial towns Fort Bragg has been given a rare opportunity to reinvent itself. I think we have an amazing foundation on which to build from. It's going to be interesting, That's why I'm here."

Sunset at Lost Coast Found
Photo © by Megan Caron

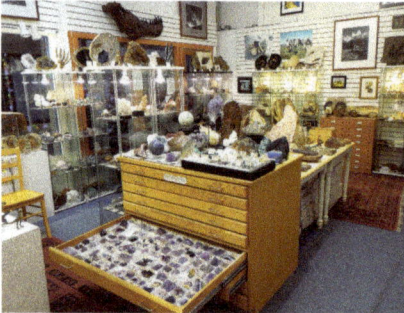

Open Wed - Sat 12-5pm, 227 East Redwood, Fort Bragg. CA 95437 (707) 364-9828

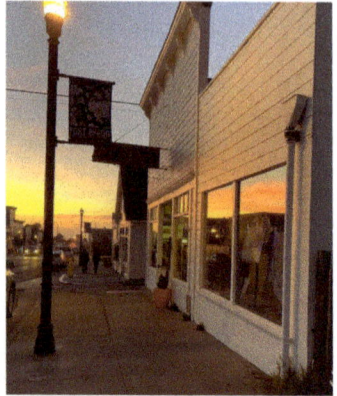

BEAUTIFUL EARTH

Gary Mason read a book about starting a rock shop in 7th grade and has been thinking about it ever since. His dream came true when he opened Beautiful Earth, a small retail shop located in the historic Railroad Depot Shopping Center. He offers minerals, fossils, meteorites, gems, stone beads, gem elixirs, and supplies. It is also a gallery for art of all media inspired by the Earth. Visitors are encouraged to ask questions, touch and talk to the rocks and explore the shop to their hearts' content. Visit the website www.beautiful-earth.net

$-$$$ BEAUTIFUL EARTH   *401 N. Main, Fort Bragg, CA. 95437*
Minerals, Fossils Art & Gifts   *Open daily 11am - 4pm*   *(707) 962-3038*

LOS GALLITOS RESTAURANT and BAR

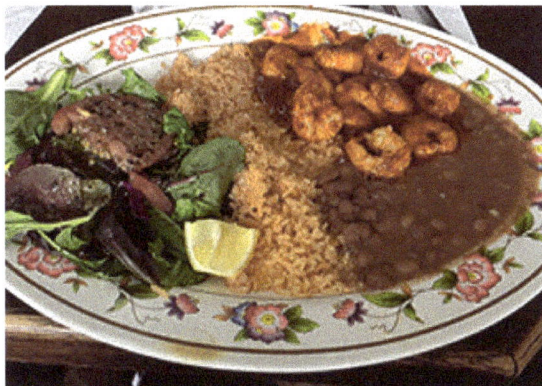

Big of heart and lengthy with menu the Valenzuela family has fed most of Fort Bragg at one time or another. The restaurant features a festive full bar and occasional live music. The fresh fish tacos are delicious. The large vegetarian burrito, with beans, rice, lettuce, cheese and salsa and the meat burrito with choice of steak, seasoned beef, chicken, marinated pork & chili verde and homemade salsa and chips are very popular. Splurge with the chili relleno and enchilada for $13.95 or the shrimp cocktails $12.75 - add octopus $3.00 more. Your proud and hard working owners are Margarita and Efrain Valenzuela and family.

$-$$ LOS GALLITOS   *223 North Franklin, Fort Bragg, CA. 95437*
Mexican Cuisine & Festive Cantina Bar   Open Sun 10am-7pm, M-F 11am-8pm,
Closed Thursday   *(707) 964-4519 Sit down or to Go*

PURITY MARKET

Since 1986 Robert and Randy Johnson have owned this neighborhood market; showcasing locally made foods as well as purchasing fresh organic fruits and vegetables whenever possible. The meat department has fresh daily cuts, fresh fish from Noyo Harbor and the shelves are lined with foods and amenities busy consumers need. Shop here and you support a local market that cares.

$-$$ PURITY MARKET   *242 N. Franklin Street, Fort Bragg, CA. 95437*
Full Service Grocery Store, Meat Dept, Fresh Produce, Health Food
Cash, Cards, Approved Cks   Open 8am - 7pm daily   (707) 964-0747

OAK MARKET and DELI

Colombi's Market, Motel and Laundromatt had been a Fort Bragg landmark for three generations; up until 2023. Today it is known as the Oak Market and Deli and has brand new owners. Different folks own the motel (now residental housing) and the laundromatt still operates. The new store owner has wisely maintained the theme of taking care of the locals and school kids. Tasty deli sandwiches, some of the best cuts of beef in town, daily homemade soup, candy and snacks and a line of basic groceries in the general store tradion of "everything for the every day need" is stocked. Hot coffee, cool beverages and friendly service keep folks coming back.

$-$$ OAK MARKET and DELI   *647 East Oak St., Fort Bragg, CA. 95437*
Full Service Grocery & Deli   *(707) 964-9274 Also Orders to Go*

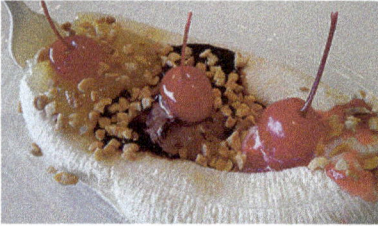

COWLICK'S ICE CREAM

Fort Bragg kids really lucked out when Cowlicks Ice Cream Parlor came to town. All their favorite ice cream sundaes and malts with delicious hot fudge, ruby red cherries, and scoops of several different varieties of ice cream are served. The famous black forest, candy cap mushroom, ginger, raspberry, strawberry and vanilla ice cream make ideal choices for that super banana split. The owners are famous for their birthday and special occasion cakes and ice cream displays. It is safer to park in the parking lot than on the street and be patient for, when the temperature hits 100 plus degrees inland, Cowlicks is inundated.

$-$$ COWLICKS   *250 N. Main Street, Suite B, Fort Bragg, CA 95437*
Gourmet Ice Cream Parlor   *Open Daily 11am to 9pm*
http://www.cowlicksicecream.com/   *(707) 962-9271 Orders to Go*

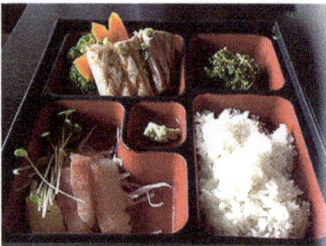

TAKA'S JAPANESE GRILL

Happy faces are on guests who have dined on Taka's sushi, tempura, teriyaki, Japanese noodle soups, and sashimi entrees. Several menus cover the numerous lunch and dinner entrees including Aukino, Oyokadan, grilled miso marinated black cod, oysters on the half shell, and chicken or beef curry rice. The wonderful Bento boxes include a choice of teriyaki chicken, beef, salmon or ahi served with choice of green salad (cucumber, seaweed or mixed greens) and miso soup with four pieces of California roll. Seating is in the cozy dining room or in the heated garden greenhouse with its lush plants. Owners Taka and Maria Takanao are living the "mom and pop" dream.

$-$$ TAKA'S JAPANESE GRILL   *250 N. Main Street, Fort Bragg, CA. 95437*
Japanese Cuisine & Bento Boxes, Beer&Wine   *Open Tues - Sun (11am to 8pm)*
See: www.northofsf.com   *(707) 964-5204 Sit down or to Go*

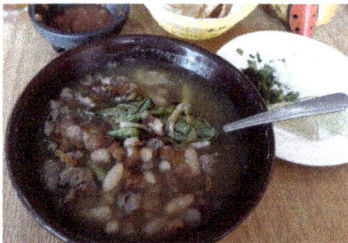

ESTRELLAS MEXICAN CUISINE

Located on Main Street next door to Taka's Japanese Grill is the popular Estrellas Mexican Restaurant. Your enthusiastic hostess is Maria Takanao. Maria loves Fort Bragg "because it is quiet and the people are so friendly". At Estrella's you can dine on authentic Mexican dishes, including chili rellenos, huevos rancheros, burritos, tacos, quesadillas, enchiladas, tamales, homemade soaps (soups) and salads. The tortillas and salsa are made fresh daily. You'll also find American dishes like hot dogs and chili dogs. Happy diners state "I was really impressed with the flavor/texture/ freshness of the food".

$-$$ ESTRELLA'S MEXICAN   *260 N. Main Street, Fort Bragg, CA. 95437*
Mexican - American Cuisine, Beer & Wine   *Open Tues-Sun 11am to 6pm*
See: www.northofsf.com   *(707) 409-5059 Sit down or to Go*

PIACI PIZZA N PUB

Proprietor Stephen Duerr has created a power-house for Pizza, Specialty Entrees and Pub Craft Beer at his popular Piaci Pub and Pizzeria in downtown Fort Bragg. The menu is simple and satisfying thin-crust piz-zas, calzone, sandwiches, salads, focaccia, baked spe-cialties using the finest in-gredients plus local & regional beer & wines. Most any day or evening of the week you'll see happy locals and visitors at this dog friendly restaurant really enjoying themselves. Nearby are ocean beaches and numerous lodges.

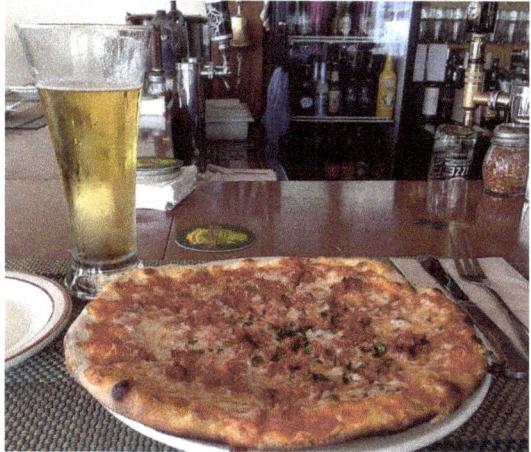

$-$$ PIACI PIZZERIA & PUB   *120 West Redwood Ave.,*
Italian - American Pizza and Brew Pub   *Fort Bragg, CA. 95437*
Open: Mon-Thur 11am - 9:30pm,   Fri & Sat till 10pm,   Sun 4 - 9:30pm
Lunch, Dinner, Full Bar, Beer & Wine,   *Cash & Debit Cards*
Sit Down, Patio Dining or Orders To Go   *(707) 961-1133*

SEA VALLEY ASIAN FUSION

Sea Valley Asian Fusion has quickly become a favorite. Located in the Com-pany Store (i.e. Lumber Mill) behind the Cookie Company you can get your fa-vorite Thai, Cambodian or Laotian food. Their green, red or yellow curry can be combined with your choice of tofu, vegetables, chicken, beef or shrimp. Green pa-paya salad comes in mild, medium or spicy hot! This is authentic cuisine sur-rounded by photographs of Fort Bragg fishing lore.

$-$$$ SEA VALLEY ASIAN FUSION 301 North Main, Fort Bragg, CA. 95437
Cambodian Laotian Cuisine   Open 4pm - 8pm (707) 200-4744 To Go Only

LEE'S CHINESE CUISINE

Lee's Chinese Restaurant has been a family tradition in Fort Bragg for more than two decades. Lee's extensive menu features classics like Mushroom Bamboo Beef, Double Kung Pao Chicken and Shrimp, Moo Goo Gaipen and much more. The Peking Dinner and Chef Lee's dinner for parties of six or more is an extrava-ganza of classic Chinese-American dishes. Catering is available as well. A rotating menu of very economical daily specials rounds out the offerings. Lee's is located on the corner of Redwood and Franklin streets in the heart of old Fort Bragg.

$-$$ LEE'S CHINESE CUISINE   154 E. Redwood Ave., Fort Bragg, CA
Mandarin Cuisine   L 11am-3pm / D 3pm-9pm,   (707) 964-6843

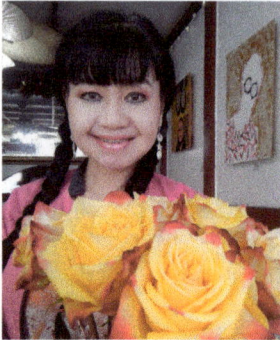

NIT'S THAI - FRENCH CAFE

Gentle beauty is a good way to describe Nit's Cafe on Main Street Fort Bragg. Nit Solmes and her French - Thai Cafe serves traditional Thai entrees with the influence of Classic French gourmet cooking. Artistic presentations of crispy spring rolls, coconut milk soup in lemongrass-galangal broth, fresh fish catch of the night, green beef curry, red chicken curry, Pad Thai and dishes with homemade fresh local and organic ingredients are served.

$-$$ NIT'S CAFE
Thai-French Cuisine   322 N. Main Street, Fort Bragg
Authentic Thai Cuisine Open Tues - Sun (11am to 8pm) Lunch, Dinner, Premium Wine & Beer (707) 964-7187 Sit down or orders to go.

MENDOCINO COOKIE COMPANY and COFFEE HOUSE

This landmark bakery coffee house has always been committed to using organic coffee beans to make their espresso, mochas and lattes. The cookies ($1.50 ea) are delicious. Varieties include chocolate chip (with or without walnuts), double fudge brownie, oatmeal raisin, ginger molasses, backpackers, peanut butter and more (ask which cookie is the special of the day).   Pastries ($3), muffins, scones, croissants. The backpacker cookie is great for camping trips. One is not enough - buy 3 or 6 to last. Thirsty? How about frozen drinks, blended frosty drinks, iced brews, Italian Soda, orange juice, organic apple juice, iced or blended mochas and iced green tea, hot chocolate, cider, milk, spring and sparkling water and lemonade. Smoothies include tropical, very berry, or strawberry banana and are nutritious and delicious (16 oz. $ 6) Come in hungry and leave happy.

$-$$ MENDOCINO COOKIE COMPANY   322 N. Main Street, Fort Bragg
Coffee, Mochas, Tea, Pastries, Cookies   Open Daily (7am to 6pm)
https://www.mendocinocookiecompany.com/ (707) 964-0282 Sit down or to go

NOYO CENTER for Marine Sciences and Natural History Museum

The Noyo Center began when a group of environmentalists wanted to create a research facility dedicated to the study and preservation of marine mammals, birds and whales. Philanthropists helped fund a showroom on Main Street Fort Bragg and the Crow's Nest, a small A-Frame exhibit and a tide pool aquarium on the Noyo Headlands. Then the Slack Tide Cafe was added in Noyo Harbor, which was formerly Carine's Italian restaurant. Research is being conducted here to bring back the kelp forests and manage sea urchins.

Interest in the Noyo Center was catalyzed when the largest whale on earth washed up in a rocky cove just south of Fort Bragg. Slowly the enormous female blue whale decomposed and workers salvaged her bone by bone. The whale sparked the idea for a larger museum to be built to house the enormous skeleton on the Noyo Headlands. Today the board, workers, volunteers and donors are raising money to build a solar powered museum large enough to exhibit the Blue Whale skeleton. Their goal is $30,000,000.

$-$$$ NOYO CENTER   Website: https://noyocenter.org/
Crow's Nest Interpretive Center: South Fort Bragg Coastal Trail (707) 733-NOYO
Discover Center Giftshop & Museum,   338 North Main, Fort Bragg, CA 95437

GUEST HOUSE MUSEUM

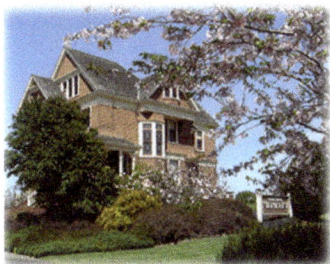

The Fort Bragg Guest House Museum was built primarily of coast redwood in 1892 by the Fort Bragg Redwood Company as a private residence. It was constructed from the finest old-growth redwood and contained 67,000 board feet of lumber. Today it is managed by the Mendocino Coast Historical Society and is full artifacts of early Fort Bragg and the Mendocino Coast. Museum hours vary, but are usually Thur-Sun from 11am-2pm. Museum staff can be reached at (707) 964-4251 and the archives at (707) 961-0498

LAUREL STREET DELI & DESSERT

Laurel Street Deli is Fort Bragg's unofficial hometown coffee shop, where a great breakfast, a hot cup, and a little lively conversation is always on the menu. Laurel Street's highly professional staff handles the large indoor-outdoor dining areas, right across the street from the Skunk Train and Guest House Museum, with speed and grace. Classic American breakfasts, a great pie selection, and chili that seems to go great with just about anything are just the beginning at Laurel Street Deli.

$-$$ LAUREL DELI & DESSERTS   *American Cuisine / Historic Museum*
401 N. Main Street, Fort Bragg, CA. 95437   *Open 6am - 4:30pm*
http://www.laureldeli.com   *(707) 964-7812 Sit down or to Go*

HEADLANDS COFFEEHOUSE

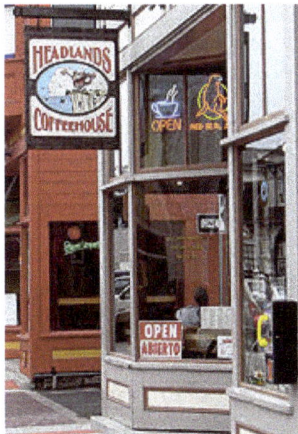

Headlands has become a go-to tradition for tourists and locals alike, right in the heart of Fort Bragg on bustling Laurel Street. Just a few steps from shops, fine food, galleries, museums, and a great jumping off point for a walk on Fort Bragg's famed coastal trail, Headlands offers a top-shelf selection of coffee drinks, plus pastries and more from local bakeries. Breakfast and lunch is served in Headlands' well-lit space, and many of the areas best musicians gather there nights for some truly mind-blowing performances and jam sessions. Packaged coffee and a constantly changing selection of art from the Mendocino Coast and beyond is also among the surprises Headlands Coffeehouse holds in store. Open daily from 8am to 8pm.

$-$$ HEADLANDS COFFEEHOUSE
Live entertainment, art & music, baked goods, entrees, soups, espresso, WiFi
120 Laurel St., Fort Bragg, CA. 95437
http://www.headlandscoffeehouse.com
(707) 964-1987 Sit Down or Orders To Go

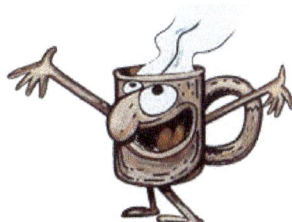

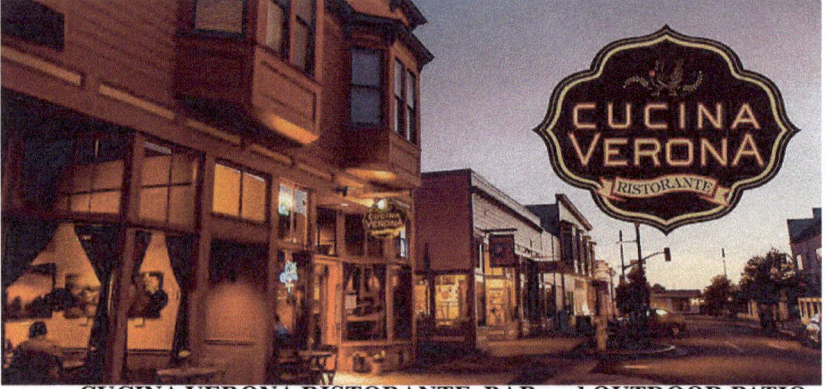

CUCINA VERONA RISTORANTE, BAR and OUTDOOR PATIO

Cucina Verona is located in the Historic Downtown District of Fort Bragg. Cucina Verona Ristorante, sports bar and outdoor patio feature Northern Italian cuisine with a Northern Californian flare. The extensive fine dining menu, created by Chef Joe Harris, includes locally caught fish and seafood, organic grass-fed beef, free-range chicken, Cioppino, pastas, fresh salads, desserts, as well as many gluten free and vegetarian options. There is a full bar, an extensive Italian wine list, and locally brewed beers on tap.

The new outdoor Patio is heated, pet friendly and is comfortable for larger groups and families with children. In the Patio kitchen, Sorrento style pizzas are made in wood fired ovens, as well as lasagna, soups, salads, burgers and sandwiches.

Espressos, lattes and pastries are made fresh daily in the adjoining Cucina Verona Mercato (a unique Italian specialty food and wine market), located at 353 North Franklin Street. Here you can purchase snacks to go, picnic goodies or authentic Italian gourmet foods for home or work. Cucina Verona is a favorite of locals and travelers alike who are looking for an excellent dining experience. Open for lunch 11:30-3pm, dinner 5:00pm-9pm, tuesday through saturday with sunday brunch 9am-3pm   Reservations are suggested.

$-$$ CUCINA VERONA	*124 East Laurel, Street,*
California - Italian Cuisine / Full Bar	*Fort Bragg, CA. 95437*
Cash, Approved Cks & Credit Cards	*(707) 964-6844 Res Advised*
Also CUCINA VERONA MERCATO	*http://www.cucinaverona.com*

EGGHEAD'S RESTAURANT

Like a long narrow sliver of pie, the Egghead's Restaurant is sandwiched between two main street buildings in downtown Fort Bragg. Furnished with corner tables and spacious booths (seating for 36) the decor is a Wizard of Oz theme. The aromas of prepared from scratch omelettes, benedicts, many unique specialties, fresh brewed coffee and espresso spills out into the dining room. Vegetarian or heart healthy choices, pancakes, egg dishes, homemade salsa and hollandaise as well as fresh squeezed juice, fresh salads, unusual sandwiches and 1/2 lb burgers are served.

$-$$ EGGHEAD OMELETTES of OZ	*Established in 1976*
Country Breakfast and Lunch	*326 N. Main Street, Fort Bragg, CA. 95437*
Open 7 days a week (7am to 2pm)	*"Toto" to go orders (707) 964-5005*

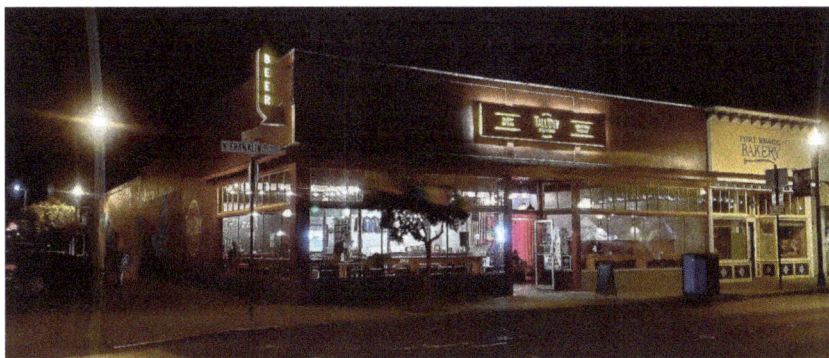

TALL GUY BREWING "If you want the beer. You gotta get it here"

Tall Guy Brewing is quite the social headquarters where visitors and Mendocino Coast residents gather to drink, dine and plan fun to serious events in their life. Located in the very heart of Fort Bragg, this spacious dining hall is child, pet and family friendly. Fourteen custom made on the premises craft beers, root beer and soda await your taste buds.

They include HAZA MAMA IPA with heavy tropical and citris aromas from heavy doses of late hops to the whirlpool and multiple doses of dry hops to the fermenter. The classic hazy hops, Citra and Mosaic, are joined by Roy Farms Azacca and Australia's Galaxy hops. MUNOZ ESPECIAL is a Mexican-style lager, which is light-bodied, light-lagger brew, MUST BE HELLES is a classic Bavarian Helles, brewed with 100% imported German malts & hops. SLEEPY LONDON PORTER is a classic English-style porter brewed with 100% imported UK malts & hops. GUNGA DENNY IPA is a 90's-era IPA. A big, amber ale at with a whopping dose of bitterness, GIMME SELTZER is a hard seltzer which can be taken straight or with a shot of Toriani-brand fruit syrup. SOFT SELTZER is a non-alcoholic seltzer. Plain or with a shot of Toriani-brand fruit syrup of your choice: Blackberry, Raspberry, Strawberry, Cherry, Pomegranate, Lime & Sugar-Free Blueberry.

As far as food options, the sky is the limit. Try the Tall Man's Braggel Dog with sausage from Roundman's Smokehouse in a fresh baked Fort Bragg Bakery soft Bavarian Pretzel - great with craft beer. You can visit the Food+Merch area for in house snacks and restaurant delivery options which include Cucina Verona across the street offerng Italian entrees, fresh seafood, garden fresh salads and homemade soups. Hucks Slider House is here on Fridays and Saturdays and Carnitas Costa Rican Cuisine is served Tuesday thru Thursday. Mountain Mikes Pizza delivers mouth watering feasts and Bernillos Pizza a block to the south offers pizza, calzone and gourmet entrees. Enjoy!!

$-$$ **TALL GUY BREWING** *362 N. Franklin St, Fort Bragg 95437*
Craft Beer, Meeting Areas & Live Entertainment   (707) 964-9132
Open Sun-Fri 2pm-10pm, Sat 1pm-10pm   WiFi password: brewbeer23

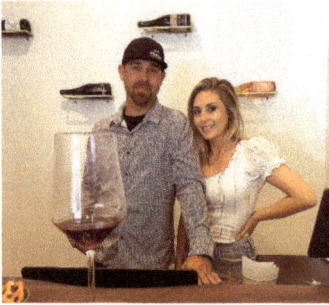

SIP WINE BAR

This cozy Wine Bar is located in the heart of Fort Bragg and is surrounded by restaurants, up scale boutiques and art galleries. The tasting room offers comfortable seating at custom redwood heart tables or the old growth long bar. Your gracious proprietress is Mahkayla Raudio.

To begin your tasting adventure you are issued a card from your host. You can taste the wines, get a half glass or full glass and taste up to 8 vintages daily at the self - serve dispensary. Delicious cheeses, meats and light snacks are in the exhibition cooler. Mendocino's finest wines are served, some created from organic and biodynamically grown grapes. Toast your life and visit to the Mendocino Coast at this truly comfortable Sip Wine Bar.

$$-$$$ SIP WINE BAR

Premium Mendocino Wines & Craft Beer   *Open Daily 11am - 5pm*
142 Laurel Street, Fort Bragg, CA 95437   *Telephone (707) 472-7092*

THE BOOKSTORE

The Bookstore is a charming mom and pop owned bookstore located in the very heart of Fort Bragg. Visitors will find a wide selection of new and used books. You can also browse through vintage vinyl. Grab a book, read, learn and relax. Local artwork is also featured. Looking to trade some of your old favorites for some new reading material? The Bookstore also buys used books. Coffee shops, restaurants, brewerys and wine tasting is across the street.

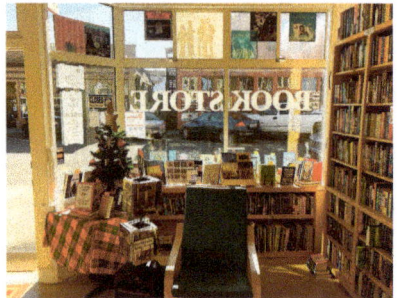

$-$$$ THE BOOKSTORE   *Open M-Sat 10:30am-5pm and Sun 11am-4pm*
New & Used Books, Vinyl   *137 E Laurel Street, Fort Bragg (707) 964-6559*

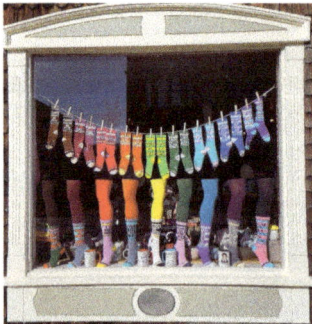

PIPPI'S SOCKS

Pippi's Longstockings is a fun whimsical casual wear boutique where every color and style of socks, striped, dotted & plaid; baby to adult; cushy, soft & feel-good to wear is stocked. Gloves, hats, handbags and sunglasses are also sold. The cheery and colorful inventory is divided into Women's Socks, Men's Socks, Women's Tights, Kids, Toe Socks, Arm & Leg Warmers, Pippi's Picks, Long Socks, Wool Socks, Foot Trafic Socks, K-Bell Socks, Ozone Socks, SmartWool Socks and Wigwam Socks. Super cushie and comfortable SmartWool socks are some of the best socks around.

$-$$ PIPPI'S SOCKS   *Socks That Make Your Feet Feel Good*
123 E. Laurel St, Fort Bragg   *Open 11am-6pm Tues-Sat*
https://www.pippisocks.com   *pippi@pippisocks.com*   *(707) 964-8071*

GLASS FIRE ART GALLERY

Eyes light up in the glow of the jelly fish sculptures frozen in glass, bowls colored like brilliant sunsets and the unique lumerian chandeliers displayed at the Glass Fire Gallery south of Fort Bragg. Artist, Buster Dyer and wife Trish built the gallery and working studio in 2005 to showcase art glass and the works from various artists including vessels, sculptures, jewelry and lighting. They look forward to hearing from you regarding your custom or commercial lighting needs.

$$-$$$ GLASS FIRE ART GALLERY

Fine Art Glass Sculpture   *(707) 962-9420*
18320 North Coast Hwy 1, Fort Bragg, CA 95437
Open 10am-5pm   *Next to the Botanical Gardens*

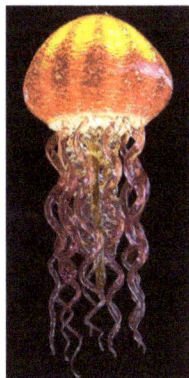

NORTHCOAST ARTISTS GALLERY

When the hearts and souls of small groups of artists gather around the campfire of imagination they inspire each other to action and manifest. Such is the case when enterprising artists met in the winter of 1986 to begin realizing a dream - to create a showroom and retail space for locally made art. The Northcoast Artists Gallery has showcased the work of 20 of Mendocino's most talented heart-centered artists for 30 years. You can experience a rare opportunity to meet the sometimes shy and reclusive to flamboyant artists, who work in the gallery and experience that their and your possibilities are absolutely endless.

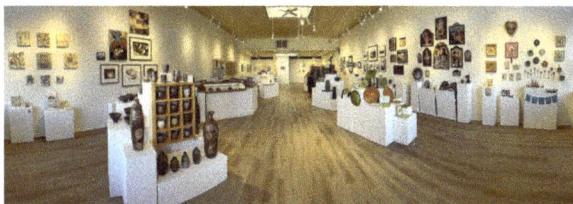

$-$$$ NORTHCOAST ARTISTS GALLERY

Artist Cooperative   *362 N. Main St., Fort Bragg, CA. 95437*
www.northcoastartists.org   *Open 10am to 5pm daily*   *(707) 964-8266*

EDGEWATER GALLERY

Edgewater Gallery is an artist-owned cooperative that opened its doors in 2003. The gallery features locally created fine art including, watercolors, oils, acrylics, photography, assemblage, ceramics, fine woodwork, jewelry, mixed media, and sculpture. They are always open to new artists joining the gallery. Both 2D and 3D artists are encouraged to apply to become guest or full-time members. Don't miss First Friday's Featured Artist presentations each month for inspiration and education.

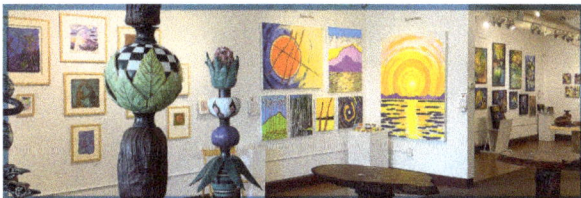

$-$$$ EDGEWATER GALLERY

Artist Cooperative   *356 N. Main St., Fort Bragg, CA. 95437*
www.edgewatergallery.com   *Open 11am to 5pm daily*   *(707) 964-8266*

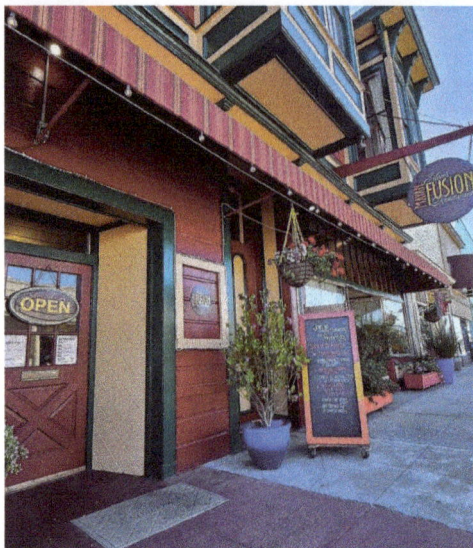

MAYAN FUSION

Award winning chef Silver Canul has created a festive showplace in the heart of Fort Bragg where he serves delicious California - South American cuisine. Mayan Fusion dishes are colorful, fresh and healthy - a dining experience you will not want to miss.

Silver is a complicated, but grounded artist who grew up on the Yucatan Peninsula from simple beginnings. He grew up immersed in the vibrant culinary and cultural traditions of his Indigenous Mayan ancestors, family, and community members. In California on the Mendocino Coast he become famous and very successful.

Mayan Fusion, which is known for its lovingly prepared dishes that showcase the best of Californian produce, meats, and seafood while featuring a fusion of spices, flavors, and techniques from Silver's rich culinary heritage and influences. Lunch selecions include enchiladas verda, burritos, coconut prawns and the delcious Thai burrito. For dinner you can enjoy Silver's award winning Cioppino, chili rellenos, fietas and osso bosso. The cozy dining room of Mayan Fusion is where neighbors can stop and chat with each other, couples can snuggle into booths for two, best-friend reunions, or you can grab a great meal in the middle of the workweek.

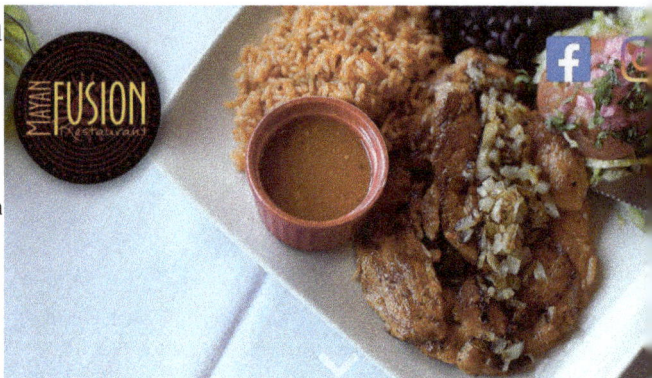

From the full bar you can order white, red and sparkling wines, plus tequila & mezcal, gin, vodka, brandy, rum, liqueurs, imported and domestic beers, ciders and non alcoholic drinks. Coffees, lattes, mochas, sparkling waters, and teas and are also served .

Sheltered under a large tent is casual patio dining. His beautifully spiced and vibrantly composed Mayan dishes like grilled Fish Tacos with Habanero Salsa Fresca, Ceviches, and his now-famous Coastal Salad, had tourists and locals alike clamoring for seats. The chowder is original and award winning. As we said, Mayan Fusion is a dining experience you will not want to miss in historic Fort Bragg.

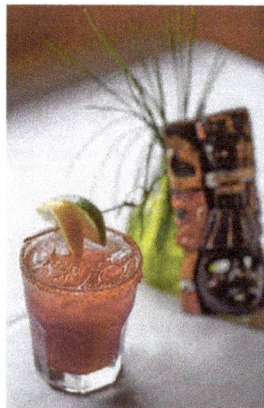

$-$$ MAYAN FUSION
A Fusion of California - South American Cuisine
Open: Monday - Sunday 11 am - 3:30 pm, 5 pm - 8:30 pm
418 N Main Street • Fort Bragg, California
https://www.mayanfusion.com/   (707) 961-0211

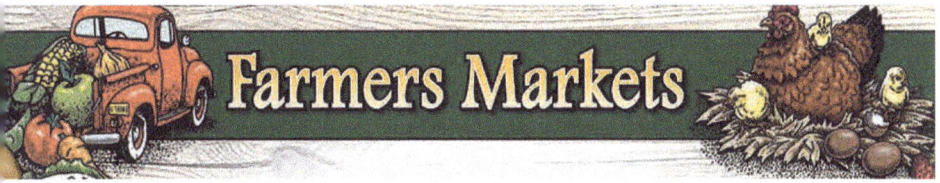
Farmers Markets

Visit Mendocino Farms at https://mcfarm.org

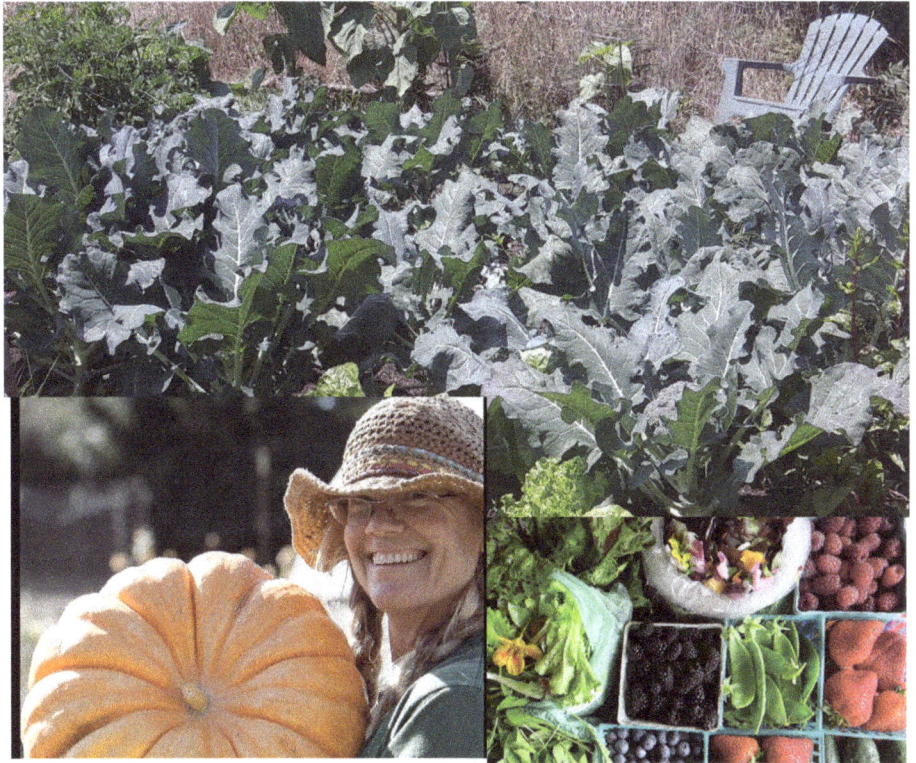

The Mendocino Farmer's Markets, which meet in Mendocino and Fort Bragg, feed 1,000s of needy residents & visitors. You can visit the Fort Bragg McFarm market on Wednesdays all year long in downtown Fort Bragg at the junction of Laurel and Franklin (May - Oct 2:30 - 5:30 and Nov - April 2:30 - 4:30). The oceanview Mendocino McFarm market meets Fridays noon to 2:30 from May - Oct at the base of Howard Street. Mendocino County is blessed with a large number of 2 - 10 acre farms which grown fruits, vegetables, herbs, medicinal plants and flowers using organic - GMO free starts. Dedicated growers such as Sakina Bush of Sakina's Gardens provided the starts for the brocolli, salad greens and fresh fruit and vegetables pictured above.

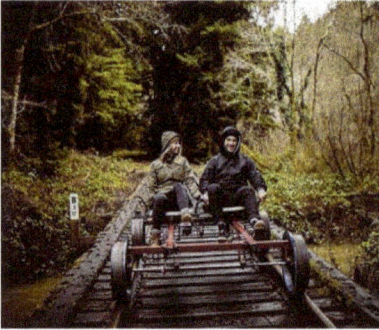

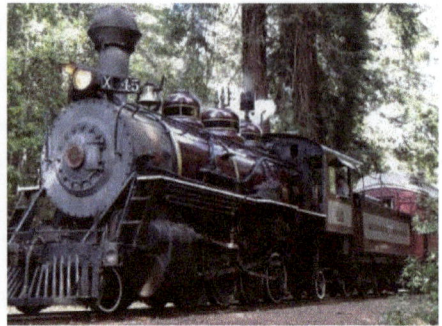

Since 1885 the historic Skunk has made its way through old-growth redwood groves, over scenic trestle bridges and through spectacular tunnels. Today the train goes west from Willits and 3 1/2 miles east from Fort Bragg into the redwoods. There is a new way to explore this same route up close and personal. The Railbike experience. Electric-powered and virtually silent, custom-built, two-person railbikes will take you breezing along this world-famous Redwood Route and into the Noyo River Canyon. You can make reservations for the train or bike by visiting https://www.skunktrain.com/

ROUNDMAN'S SMOKEHOUSE

Roundman's Smokehouse grew out of the strong fishing and hunting traditions on the Mendocino Coast and they're still available for processing or smoking deer or elk. For those interested in just a taste of Noyo salmon or some fine Humboldt County cheese, Covelo grass-fed beef, smoked duck, smoked salmon or some imaginative condiments and sauces. Don't forget about the special dog snacks in the cooler. Roundman's has that too. Located near the heart of town on Main Street, Roundman's Smokehouse is truly a taste of old Fort Bragg.

$-$$ ROUNDMAN'S   *412 North Main Street, Fort Bragg, CA. 95437*
Fresh Cuts of Meat, Smoked Salmon, Dog Bones and Deli Sandwiches
Open Daily from 10am - 5pm   *Cash, Credit Cards*   *(707) 964-5954*

MENDOCINO CHOCOLATE COMPANY

At both locations of the Mendocino Chocolate Company delicious artisanal chocolate and handmade gifts are created daily in their candy kitchen. There is an amazing selection of fresh gourmet chocolate. Signature truffles and originals, fudge and confections are handmade and decorated in small batches using the best premium ingredients and original recipes for exceptional quality and taste. To find the perfect gift you can browse on line or in person through their selection of chocolate gift boxes, novelty items, or holiday items – all made to bring that touch of coastal charm to your special recipient. Choose from sugar free, confectionary and cakes or "cookie in the crate".

$-$$ MENDOCINO CHOCOLATE COMPANY   *Open daily 11am - 5:30pm*
Homemade Chocolates, Candies & Cakes https://www.mendochocolateco.com/
IN FORT BRAGG: 410 North Main, Fort Bragg, CA. 95437   *(707) 964-8800*
IN MENDOCINO: 45050 Main Street, Mendocino, CA 95460   *(707) 937-1107*

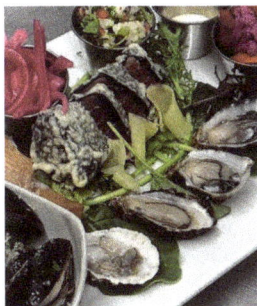

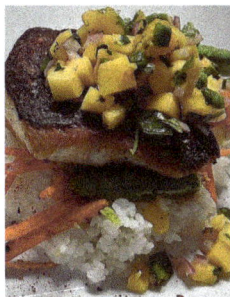

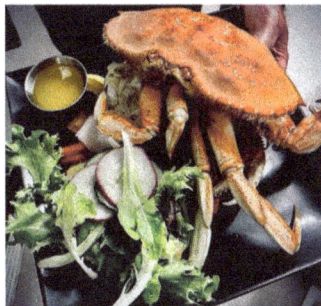

KW SALTWATER GRILL

Some locals say this upscale restaurant is the finest restaurant in Fort Bragg. Owner Kristy Wilson certainly did a beautiful job remodeling the dining room and outdoor patio with fire pits making it a truly romantic setting. The cuisine is all local wild caught fish, high quality pasture raised beef and organic produce from local farms. The fresh oysters are from the pristine Pacific Northwest.

You can begin your dining experience with the oyster sampler platter, followed by the "Little Gem Salad", or smoked seafood chowder followed by a main course. Entrees include the Saltwater Grill Cioppino, pan roasted Halibut, local caught Black Cod or grilled "bone in" Rib Steak. Devine deserts include lemon cream brue, cheese cake or chocolate hazelnut semifreddo. Plan on spending $100 per person for a 5 course dinner.

Kirsty and her experienced staff also cater weddings, special events, conventions and group meetings with exception wine lists and cuisine.

$$-$$$ KW SALTWATER GRILL   *542 N Main St, Fort Bragg, CA 95437*
Fresh wild caught seafood and choice cuts of meats. Open 5 - 9pm Tues - Sun
https://kw-saltwater-grill.squarespace.com/ (707) 900-1667 Res. Suggested

NORTH COAST BREWERY, RESTAURANT and GIFTSHOP

The North Coast Brewery was founded by liberal beer drinking New Yorkers in 1988. It has grown to produce over 70,000 barrels of beer per year. Several popular craft beers are distributed coast to coast including Scrimshaw, Old Rasputin and Prankster.

All American food is served in the restaurant - fish n chips, cheese burgers with thick cut garlic fries, fresh tossed green salads, clam chowder and the fresh fish catch of the day. A surprisingly good line-up of entertainers and musicians perform here on weekends.

$-$$ NORTH COAST BREWING COMPANY 444 North Main, Fort Bragg,
American Craft Beer / California Cuisine Live Entertainment (707) 964-3400

CAFE ONE

Cafe One is an organic breakfast and lunch choice with an international array of entrees. The menu items are "chemical-free" and non genetically modified. A colorful array of fresh local organic fruits, vegetables, herbs, meats and wild caught fish is served. Wines made from organically grown grapes, local micro-brewed beers, organic juices (fresh squeezed orange juice weekends), fair trade and organic coffee to drink. The early morning smell of oven fresh scones, just baked pies and cakes create fond memories.

$-$$ CAFE ONE   *753 N. Main Street, Fort Bragg, CA.95437*
California Organic Cuisine   MC, Visa & Approved Cks   (707) 964-3309

TRAVEL NOTES

THE WORLD FAMOUS GLASS BEACH

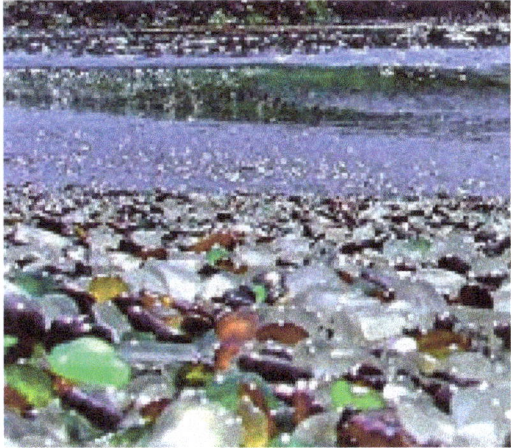

At the end of Elm Street in Fort Bragg is the world famous Glass Beach. There is no admission and folks travel here from all over the world looking for treasure. For years it was a dump or "trash beach". First horse and buggy; then residents would back their pick-up trucks to the edge of the cliff and unload their trash. Fire would burn away anything that wasn't enduring.   The ocean would flush, rush and crush the contents; each tide and storm would reduce the rubble. What remains today are little pieces of broken glass of various colors and sizes; some very rare and valuable. This is Glass Beach. The Sea Glass Museum, in the historic Union Lumber Company Store, is a great place to explore the history of Glass Beach and purchase a souvenir of rare treasure collected by sea glass and Glass Beach expert Captain Cass Forrington. His museum is a must see in Fort Bragg.

The symbology of Glass Beach is expressed by local minister Greg Esher of Grace Church, a place of worship and "hubs and routes" emergency shelter for the less fortunate. Greg states "God can take the trash of your life and His refining turbulent love can wash the filth away, deposit it in the deepest part of the ocean never to be seen again. He can carry away the pain as far as the "east is from the west" and your life will be changed from trash to treasure, your mess into a message, your test into testimony, your stumbling block into a stepping stone, and your brokenness into blessings."

Glass Beach Jewelry's Sea Glass Museum is a *"Must See"* for all ages! Showcasing the beautiful treasure of a local former sea captain who scours Fort Bragg's plentiful Glass Beaches for rare gems. The gallery also offers fine handcrafted sea glass jewelry and art. Listed on Trip Advisor as the most popular privately owned attraction on the coast.

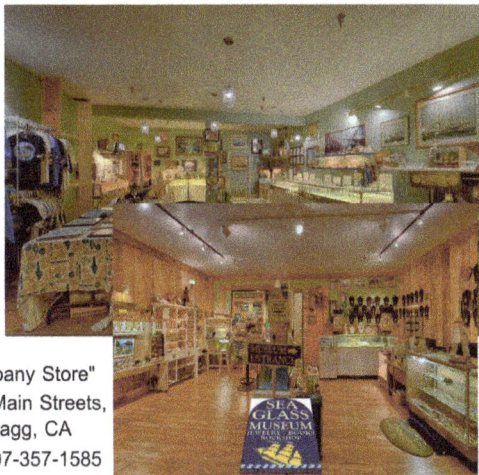

Located in the Historic "Company Store" at the corner of Redwood & Main Streets, 303 N. Main St., Ste F, Ft. Bragg, CA
GlassBeachJewelry.com - 707-357-1585

NELLO'S MARKET

Located on the north end of Fort Bragg a few blocks from the world famous Glass Beach is Nello's Market. Nellos has been a popular neighborhood market since the 50's with locals and serves up some amazing sandwiches and gourmet entrees. Besides the food there is the liquor, potato chips, candy bars and nonalcoholic drinks from A-Z. Nello's is open daily and service is fast at this usually very busy store. Parking is awkward so be careful pulling in and out as locals in big trucks get impatient.

$-$$ NELLO'S MARKET   860 N. Main Street, Fort Bragg, CA. 95437
Delicatessen, Groceries, Beer & Wine, Picnic Supplies, Delicious Sandwiches
Cash, Cards & Approved Cks   Open 8am - 8pm daily   (707) 964-2007

BEACHCOMBER MOTEL, BEACH HOUSE INN, HARBOR LITE LODGE, SURF n SAND and The WHARF RESTAURANT

Located at the north end of Fort Bragg near the Pudding Creek trestle are properties owned by the Beachcomber Hotel Group; the Beach House Inn overlooking Pudding Creek, the Beachcomber Motel, Surf n Sand Motel on the beach and south by the Noyo River bridge, the Harbor Lite Lodge. A large variety of rooms and suites with king, queen and double beds, private baths, cable TVs and some with kitchenettes await. Some of the luxury suites have indoor hot tubs. Children love the peaceful adventure of racing the bluffs and trails and then returning to their safe and cozy room. Seasonal rates are from $99 to $259/2 per night. While wintertime gale force winds and the elements are orchestrating a magnificent show outside, you can be bubbling away in your private hot tub with a cheery fire crackling in the fireplace.

$$ BEACHCOMBER MOTEL   1111 North Main, Fort Bragg, CA. 95437
Oceanviews, Fireplaces, Hot Tubs, In-room coffee makers, refrigerators, cable
color TV's & free WiFi.   https://www.thebeachcombermotel.com/
(707) 964-2402   Toll Free: 1-800-400-SURF (7873) Reservations
$$ BEACH HOUSE INN   100 Pudding Creek Road, Fort Bragg, CA. 95437
Ocean & Beach View Motel Rooms & Suites   (707) 961-1700 Res. Advised
$$-$$$ HARBOR LITE LODGE 120 N. Harbor Drive Fort Bragg, CA. 95437
Rooms & Suites   http://www.harborlitelodge.com (707) 964-0221 Res. Advised
$$-$$$ SURF and SAND LODGE   1131 North Main, Fort Bragg, CA. 95437
Motel Rooms & Suites http://www.surfnsand.com (707) 964-9383 Res. Advised

BEST WESTERN VISTA MANOR LODGE

Set on coastal bluffs overlooking pristine ocean beaches and the Pudding Creek trestle is the Vista Manor Lodge. Spacious accommodations include 54 remodeled rooms with natural wood, bright colored carpets, drapes, bedspreads, private baths, cable TV and in-room telephones. Optional continental breakfast is served in the common room adjacent the lobby and heated olympic swimming pool. A two bedroom cottage complete with a kitchen and fireplace is ideal for small conferences or social gatherings. Room rates are from $125 summertime, and $95 wintertime; the cottage is from $225 per day.

$$-$$$ BEST WESTERN VISTA MANOR   1100 North Main,
Motel Rooms & Suites   Fort Bragg, CA. 95437
http://www.bwfortbragg.com   (707) 964-4776 Res. Advised

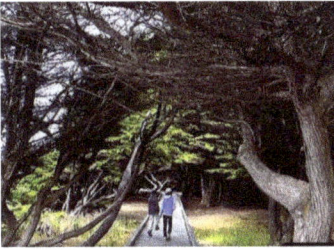

MacKERRICHER STATE PARK

Mac Kerricher is the gemstone of Mendocino Coast State Parks; located five miles north of Fort Bragg in the tiny community of Cleone (Portuguese for "gracious people"). Each of the park's 142 family campsites, which can accommodate tents or recreational vehicles up to 35 feet long, has a stove, table, and cupboard with piped water nearby. Rates are $45 per site/per night - 2 cars - 8 people max. Combination buildings with hot showers, restrooms and laundry facilities are available. Across the highway is Richochet Ridge Horse Ranch which offers trail rides to the beach. The horses are gentle and trail rides a wonderful way to connect with nture. For trail rides you can call (707) 964-7669 or visit 24201 N. Hwy 1, Fort Bragg   Richocheet Ridge Ranch website is https://www.horse-vacation.com

$$ MacKERRICHER STATE PARK Overnight Camping 1 vehicle $45/night
Reservations 1-800-444-PARK   https://www.parks.ca.gov/?page_id=436

CLEONE GROCERY STORE
CAMPGROUND & GAS STATION

Behind the full service grocery store and gas station is a lush campground with bathrooms, hot showers, a laundry room, fish cleaning facility and garbage pick-up. A coastal breeze nudges tree tops and bows into motion as you tend your open pit fire in the windbreak below. It feels good to camp here, especially knowing that the clean and well organized store, scarcely100 feet away, is there to provide for all your basic camping needs. The full service store and gas station stocks lots of frozen meals, some fresh produce, milk, cheese, sandwich meats, ice cream, a good selection of beer and premium wines, camping equipment, toiletries, soaps, cooking utensils and campfire fuel.

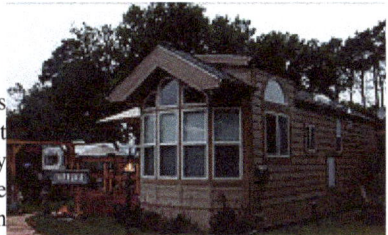

The 36 campsites on 5 acres in this peaceful oceanside setting are set under a forest canopy with hedgerows and landscaping providing privacy and natural beauty. Pull through and RV sites offer campfire rings, picnic tables, water and electricity. Overnight rates are very fair and camp rules are enforced for peace and safety. Bring your friends, children and pets for a wonderful vacation in Cleone.

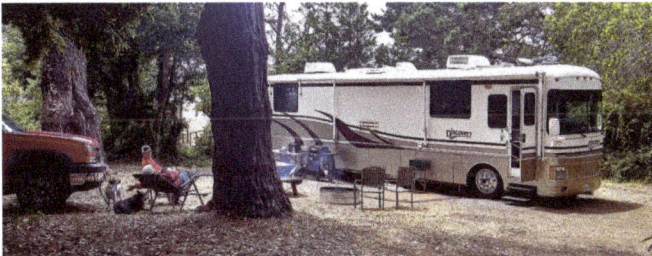

$-$$ CLEONE GROCERY & CAMPGROUND   24400 N. Hwy 1, Cleone
Campground, Full Service Grocery Store & Gas Station, Hot Showers
Store & Gas Open 7:30am-9pm   http://www.cleonecampground.com/
Seasonal Campground   Res. Nec. (707) 964-4589   Store (707) 964-2707

INN at NEWPORT RANCH

The Inn at Newport Ranch is an extraordinary property that exemplifies the restorative power of nature. The ranch is set like a gemstone above the Pacific Ocean with open meadow vistas beneath a three mile ridge line of redwood forests teaming with wildlife. Guests can opt to stay in suites in the Main Inn Building, the Redwood House Suites, the Ranch House, Barb's Place or the luxurious Sea Drum Oceanfront Home. Amenities are too numerous to mention here, but a few include a walk-in fireplace and a rooftop hot tub - see amenities on website. Rates start at $900 (Ridgeview Room). Pictured above is the main lodge and restaurant. Greatness can be manifested here.

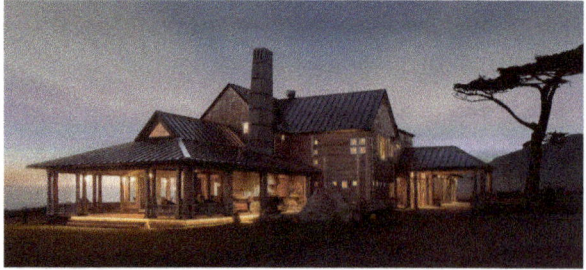

Elevated Ranch Cuisine is served to Inn guests breakfast, lunch and dinner and "friends of the Ranch." The culinary team cook over live fire sourcing materials from the ranch and local environs that result in amazing flavor profiles. There is a stunning spa where guests can receive life promoting treatments of massage, hydro therapy, medicinal herbs and crystal clear air. Sleeps are deep with the sounds of the wind and crashing surf beneath a starlit sky. The Inn at Newport Ranch is a great destination for groups, weddings, yoga workshops or for reconnecting with nature and your creator.

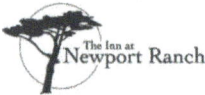

$$$ THE INN AT NEWPORT RANCH

Luxury Resort; To Reserve & Additional Information   *(707) 962-4818*
https://www.theinnatnewportranch.com/ 31502 N. Hwy 1, Fort Bragg, 95437

SWITZER FARM WEDDINGS

Switzer Farm is one of the most majestic and secluded wedding destinations on California's Coast. Located 20 minutes north of Fort Bragg and just south of Westport, the 1884 restored Victorian farmhouse sits atop 22 oceanfront acres directly above the wild Pacific. The farm is completely private. There is nothing between you and the ocean but a very private meadow, headlands and coastal cliffs. To the delight of guests the flower gardens attract angelic flutters of butterflies and humming birds. Owner Gary Weiss is proud of the many magical weddings and varied venues he has hosted here. Wedding cost $23,000 /3 nights up to 99 guests.

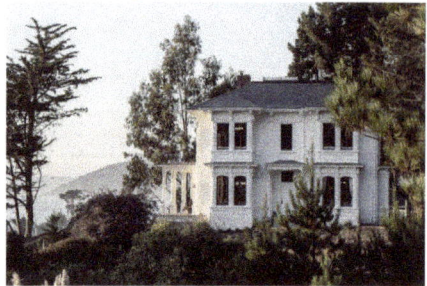

Photo by Freda Banks

$$-$$$ SWITZER FARM   *36700 N. Hwy 1, Westport, CA. 95437*
Weddings, Lodging and Reception Destination   *(707) 409-0383*
https://switzerfarm.com/   *gary@switzerfarmofwestport.com*

WESTPORT HOTEL
and Old ABALONE PUB

The Westport Hotel is a historic Victorian Bed & Breakfast (circa 1890) located on Highway 1 at Westport. Upstairs are six comfortable rooms with private baths and ocean views. The inn can accommodate couples or groups of up to 12 people with standard rates for 2 from $243 - $303; whale watching and ocean access is across the street.

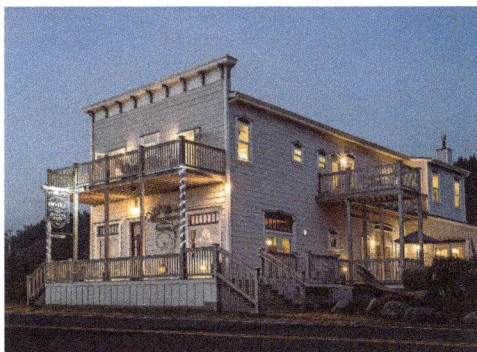

The chef uses only local catches of fish, small farm and garden organic produce and cuts of beef and chicken. Four to five special dishes are served for dinner depending on the chefs "whims and moods". The food is absolutely delicious. A variety of micro-brewed beers and California wines are served at the georgeous redwood heart bar or tableside. Of special note are Dorine's afternoon teas served on Saturday afternoons by reservation. During the logging and fishing boom of the 1800's Westport was home to 14 saloons. Only the best is left - the Westport Hotel and Old Abalone Pub.

$$-$$$ WESTPORT HOTEL   *38921 N. Hwy. 1, Westport, CA 95488*
Bed n Breakfast/Dinners, Old Abalone Pub, Beer and Wine Bar, High Teas, Sauna, Jacuzzi Tubs. http://www.westporthotel.us (707) 964-3688 Res. Nec.

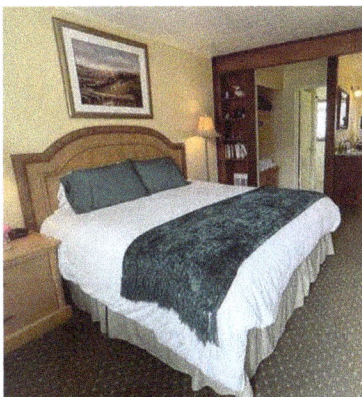

LOST COAST VISTA INN

One of the warmest motel "inns" on the north coast was the Westport Inn. The main motel was built right after World War II in 1947, with the heart of the dining room built in 1895 during the boom town days of exploding Westport! The Lost Coast Vista Inn has a new name and a new vision thanks to innkeeper /chef Tabitha Korhummel. Visitors share the cozy dining room while enjoying delicious vegetarian, snack food and delicious espresso and mochas. During winter you can relax around the living room fire and on balmy summer days the outdoor patio with the fragrance of Sutter Gold roses. Six comfortable rooms (from $150-190/2 + tax) provide tranquility and quiet except for the nearby roar of the Pacific and the wind whistling through the Westport trees.

$-$$ LOST COAST VISTA INN   *P.O. Box 145, Westport, CA 95488*
Rooms and Suites   Major Credit Cards   (707) 964-5135 Res. Advised

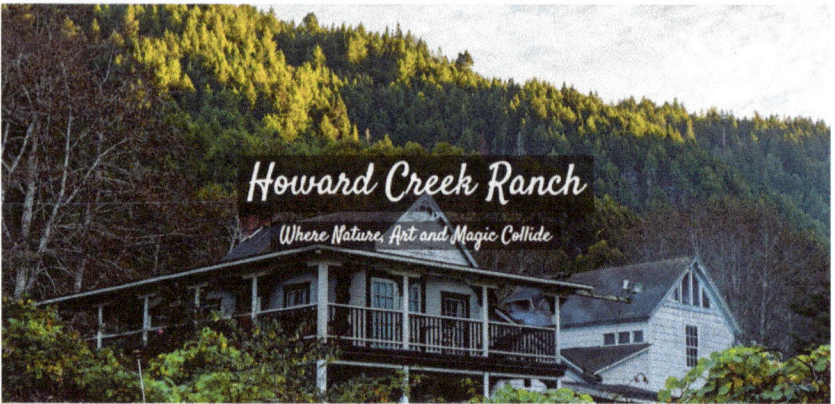

HOWARD CREEK RANCH

Award winning flower gardens, accommodations crafted from virgin redwood milled right from the ranch, sumptuous full breakfasts, indoor & outdoor spas with hot and cold pools, an array of wildlife makes this 60 acre ranch a nice vacation destination for lovers, thinkers or those seeking to heal and alleviate stress. Accommodations with ocean, creek and forest views, wood stoves, fireplaces, private baths, king and queen beds are combined with other amenities. Rates for two are from $175 - $258.

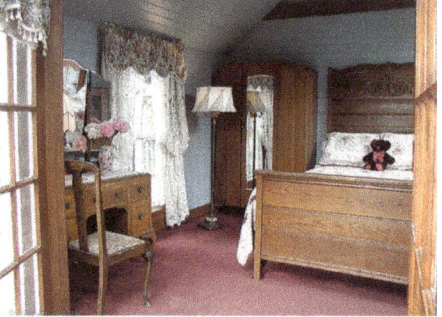

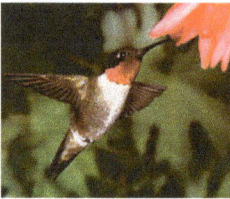

$$-$$$ HOWARD CREEK RANCH
Bed & Breakfast Ranch
All Major Credit Cards
P.O. Box 121, 40501 N. Hwy 1, Westport, CA. 95488
http:// www.howardcreekranch.com
(707) 964-6725 Reservations

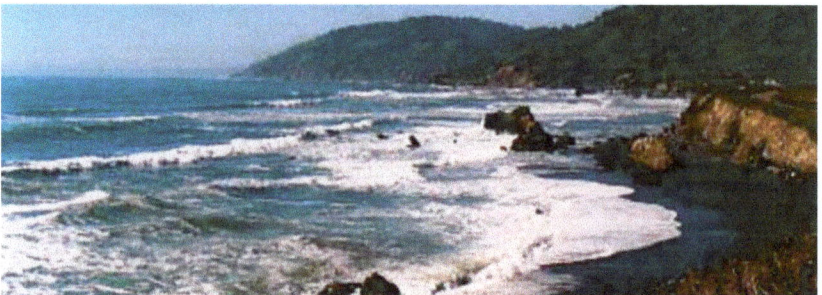

WESTPORT COMMUNITY STORE

A welcome site indeed, for those coming to/from the Lost Coast. You can count on piping hot coffee, homemade deli sandwiches, organic produce, premium wines, cool drinks, gasoline, oil and reliable information 365 days of the year. Though the store looks rustic on the outside and is only 1,000 square feet, the owners make sure there is something for all appetites. Don't forget, it's the 1st store on Route 1 from Highway 101 at Leggett and the last stop for provisions if you are headed into the Lost Coast; so check gear, gas up, get water and last minute provisions.

$-$$$ WESTPORT COMMUNITY STORE   *38921 N. Coast Hwy 1,*
General Store, Gasoline, Water, Organic Food   *Westport, CA 95488*
Cheeseburgers, Deli, Beer & Wine Open Daily 8am - 6pm   *(707) 964-2872*

WESTPORT BEACH CAMPGROUND

The Westport Beach RV Park and Campground is located at sea level just north of Westport. Though it is a nice place to spend a few days it is also is a potential kill zone if a Tsunami rolls in and licks it off the face of the earth. Visitor(s) beware, but do enjoy the sandy beach and nearby sights and sounds. Feel a major shaker? Be prepared to get yourself and loved ones up to the top of the State Highway One hill within 15 minutes (the Tsunami surge travels 600 mph and most likely will come from the north). Camping rates are $49 for the first 2, regular RV sites $65 for first 2, premium RV sites are $75.

$-$$ WESTPORT BEACH RV PARK & CAMPGROUND
Oceanside Camping, RV Hook-ups   *37700 Hwy. 1, Westport, CA 95488*
http://www.westportbeachrv.com   *(707) 964-2964 Res. Suggested*

WESTPORT—UNION LANDING STATE BEACH

For hundreds of years these headlands were the sacred hunting ground of the Pomo Indians. They caught surf fish, rock fish; gathered abalone and mussels and foraged for medicinal plants and seaweed. For decades camping was free here and loggers who worked the woods to the north and recreation vehicle families used to stay for months to fish and sleep under the stars.

But 1987 marked an end to all this. Today's campers will find picnic tables, BBQ firepits, cold running drinking water and primitive outdoor toilets for a $45 overnight camping fee (additional vehicles $10) at one of 100 prepared campsites. Sorry, no showers, more improvements are planned and there is an informative resident ranger and evening campfire talks. The Westport Union Landing State Beach offers 2 miles of ocean front with grassy meadows dotted with wildflowers, steep unstable cliffs and sandy beaches. Stabilized foot trails and terraced redwood stairways lead down to the sea. Dangerous currents, blue and great white sharks prowl the depths; so be careful with your children and pets. One diver's head was literally bitten off.

$ WESTPORT—UNION LANDING STATE BEACH
Oceanside Campground   *P.O. Box 440, Mendocino, CA 95460*
Reserve America at1-800-444-PARK   *(707) 937-5804 Res. and Info.*

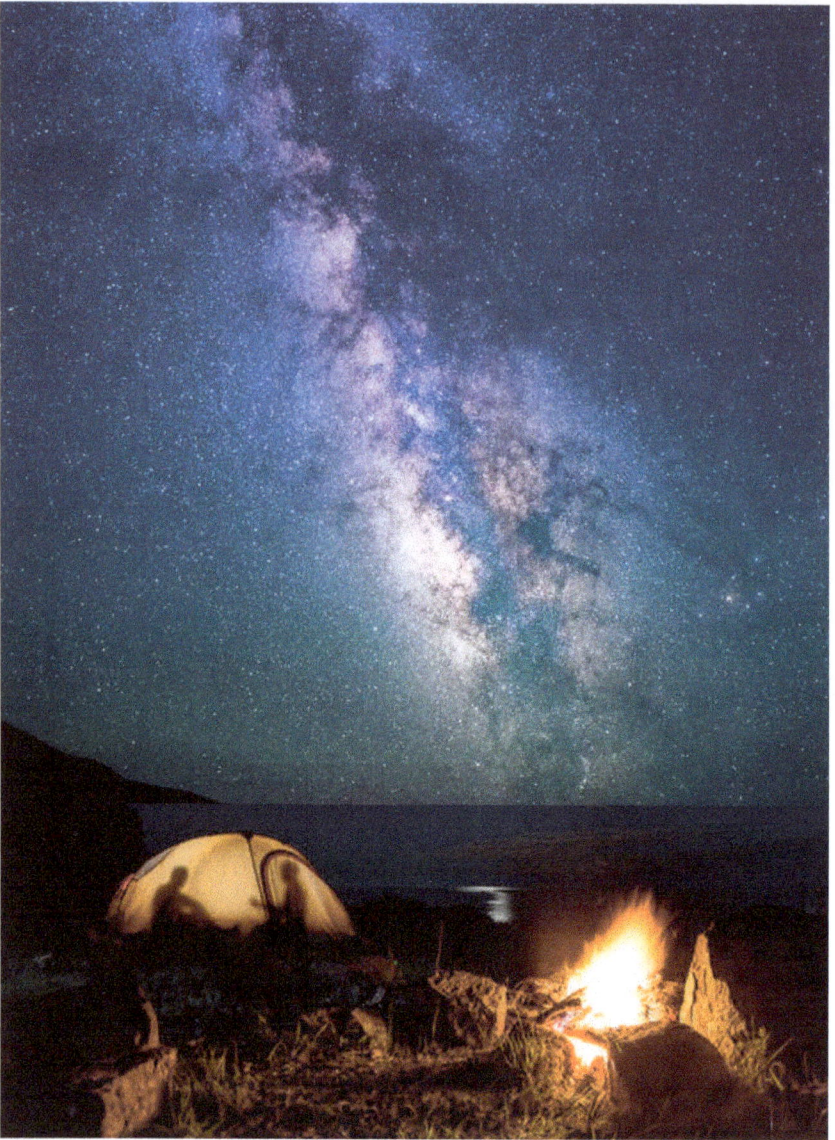

Some of your more memorable life experiences can be spent on the Lost Coast in a tent, at night with the lullaby of the waves beating against the shore and the stars overhead. Some nights are so quiet and peaceful that all you can hear is your lovers heart beating in harmony with yours. You can "shed your cloak of formality" and get real in such places. Having the proper amenities is important. I suggest you visit the Outdoor Store in Mendocino or Fort Bragg.

The Mendocino Coast Food & Shelter Safety Net You Can Support By Donation

The FORT BRAGG FOOD BANK feeds 1,000s of needy residents & visitors

Every week the kind staff at the Fort Bragg Food Bank hand out bags of fresh produce, some from local organic farms, as well as canned and packaged breakfast, lunch and dinner items. Coffee, tea, fruit juices, milk and words of encouragement mean a lot.

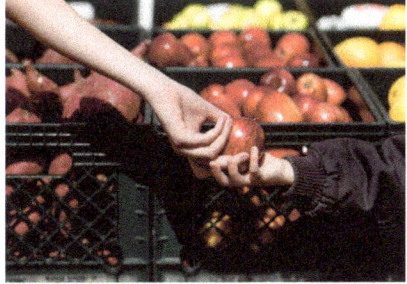

http://www.fortbraggfoodbank.org

Shockingly One in Four Mendocino Coast Children go to Bed Hungry !

Please donate to the Childrens Fund and you help end short term and long term suffering among children and their struggling families. A garden network helps provide kids with delicious home grown produce.

http://www.mccf.info/.org

Homeless People are most at risk of exposure to the elements.

The Hospitality House provides shelter for at risk and homeless people who want to work their system of rebuilding self-esteem, meaningful employment and safety. They offer 24 beds for people each night; provide meals, training and motel vouchers for more.

http://www.mendocinochc.org/

ARK GIFTSHOP for the MENDOCINO COAST HUMANE SOCIETY

At the Ark Pet Store Giftshop you can support the care and feeding of Mendocino Coast Humane Society dogs and cats by purchasing quality used merchandise. This "feel good" store is located west of the State Highway 1 round-about. The Ark Thrift Shop is the coast's premier emporium of used and recycled treasures and provides a substantial share of the money needed to keep the Shelter in operation.

18274 N. Hwy 1, Fort Bragg, CA. 95437 Open daily noon -5pm   707 961-0365

http://mendocinohumane.org/

SAFETY FROM WILDFIRES IS CRITICAL TO TOURISM

One of the most critical areas for wildfire protection is the Simpson Lane - Mitchell Creek area in south Fort Bragg. A huge fuel load build-up exists in Jughandle State Forest from an old logging cut and dereliction by California State Parks. This is one of the most densely populated areas of Mendocino County with many mom and pop business owners and Fort Bragg consumers living there. Donate to the Fort Bragg South Fire Safe Council and you help protect life, property and Fort Bragg itself from wildfire spread.

http://www.firesafefortbraggsouth.com

The Safety Net of CHURCHES
From Extraction, to Addiction, to Attraction

The Mendocino coast is ground zero for what became the world's fifth largest economy when a '49er named Jerome Ford came up to scavenge a shipwrecked Chinese schooner, the Frolic. He looked ashore and saw the real treasure and built the first lumber mill at Casper Creek. The Redwood Highway, coupled with a world-class port created the extraction economy. Forestry and fishing built an amazing community along the Pacific Ocean with the two seaport cities Fort Bragg and the village of Mendocino. With the removal of the mills and the ocean in distress we became "a drinking town with a fishing problem." Mendocino County emerged with a new economy: wine, beer, meth, marijuana, fentanyl, heroin and gambling becoming the norm.

The air conditioned Mendocino Coast, however, has much to offer with its unfettered access to the Pacific Ocean: tidal pools, gardens, ocean bluffs and sunsets. We are working to move away from the addiction economy to the attraction economy; healing hearts and minds, where people come for the beauty of creation and glory of God. Listed here are the churches serving that vision.

by Greg Escher, pastor / Grace Community Church

CHURCHES ON THE MENDOCINO COAST THAT CAN ENRICH YOUR VISIT

MENDOCINO (Zip Code 95460)

Mendocino Presbyterian Church
44831 Main St., Mendocino, CA 95460
https://www.mendopres.org/
Pastor: Mathew Davis   (707) 937-5441
Service Sunday 10:30am
Homeless Help with Food & Showers.

Mendocino Baptist Church
Little Lake St & Kasten Rd., Mendocino
https://mendocinobaptistchurch.com/
Pastor: Jim Kirby   (707) 937-5088
Service 10:30 am Sunday
Outreach and Prayer Services

COMPTCHE (Zip Code 95427)

Chapel of the Redwoods
31201 Comptche-Ukiah Rd., Comptche,
Pastor: Doug Moyer   (707) 937-0850

Saint Anthony Roman Catholic Church
10700 Lansing St., Mendocino, CA
Priest: Rob Torczynski (707) 937-5808
Service Sunday 10am

CASPAR (Zip Code 95420)

Caspar Community Center
Complete emergency supplies, equipment, solar and generator, commercial kitchen, gardens, shelter. meeting and banquet facilities.
https://casparcommons.org/

Mendocino Coast Jewish Community
15071 Caspar Rd., Caspar, CA ·
(707) 964-6146   Service 10:30 am
https://www.mcjc.org/
Rabbi: Margaret Holub

FORT BRAGG (Zip 95437)

Assamblea Apostolica De La Fe
24521 N. Highway 1 Fort Bragg
Apostolic   (707) 964-1486
Pastor: Miguel Estrella
Service Sunday 10am

Bethel Baptist Church
31200 Highway 20, Fort Bragg
Pastor: Ken Word (707) 357-0711
Service Sunday 11am

Calvary Baptist Church
1144 E. Chestnut St, Fort Bragg
Pastor: Josh Margevison
Non-Denominational
(707) 964-2366
Service Sunday 10am

Calvary Chapel Fort Bragg
900 N. Main St. Fort Bragg CA
Pastor: Kevin Green   (707) 961-6252
Service Sunday 10 am & 6:30 pm

Coast Christian Center
Assembly of God
1004 E. Chestnut St. Fort Bragg CA
Pastor: Kris Strickland (707) 964-5247
Service Sunday 11am & Wed. 6pm

Evergreen United Methodist Church
360 N. Corry St., Fort Bragg CA
Pastor: Diana Hunter (707) 964-5497
Service Sunday from 11:00 am

First Baptist Church
511 N. Franklin St. Fort Bragg CA
Pastor: Chris Aycock (707) 964-3422
Service Sunday 10:30am

First Presbyterian Church
of Fort Bragg 367 S. Sanderson Way ·
http://www.fortbraggpresbyterian.org/
Rev. Dr. John Carrick (707) 964-2316
Service Sunday 10am

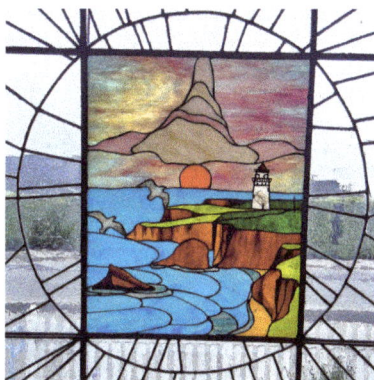

Grace Community Church
http://www.fbgracecommunitychurch.com/
1450 E Oak St. Fort Bragg
Pastor: Greg Escher   (707) 964-4107
Emergency Shelter / Hubs & Routes
Service Sunday 10am

Mendocino Center for Spiritual Living
301 N. Main Fort Bragg
https://www.mendocinocsl.org/
Rev. Tanya Wyldflower   (707) 964-1458
Service Sunday 11am Workshop Classes

Our Lady of Good Council / Catholic
255 S. Harold St. Fort Bragg CA 95437
http://www.olgcinfb.org/
Fr. Andre's L. F. Querijero, Jr.
(707) 964-0229

St. Michaels All Angels Episcopal Church
201 E. Fir, Fort Bragg, CA. 95437
Reverand: Randy A. Knutson
(707) 964-1900 Service Sunday 10am

Trinity Lutheran Church
620 E. Redwood Ave., Fort Bragg CA
Minister: Randy Knutson (707) 964-5032
Service Sunday 9am

Westport Community Church
Abalone St., Westport, CA 95488
Reserve for Talks or Seminars
erind.3500@gmail.com (707) 489-2546

TRAVEL NOTES

My Secret Hideaway

I will not tell you the secret little hideaways I have found where a thousand leaves, evergreen bows and ferns wave at me in a gentle breeze. Here the earth is very soft and fertile, the grasses like a carpet of fleece and the plant medicine very strong. I slow my heartbeat in the quietness and relax into the moment. I sense the plant spirits, watch the dragonflys, butterflys and hummingbirds dart about. Lobo is grounded here and his alertness keeps me safe. The setting is wild and could be dangerous. Every color of green is around me and I slip off into a deep sleep on this beloved planet I call home.

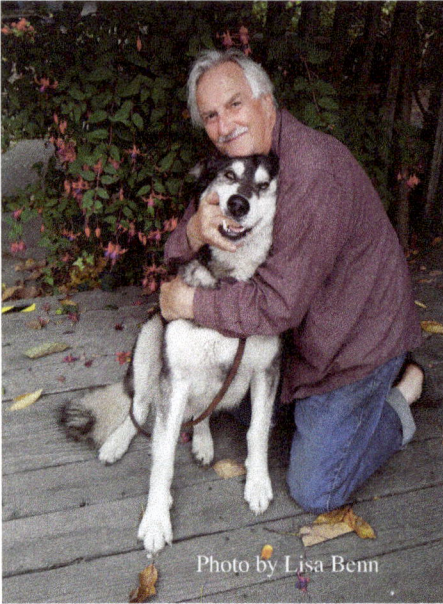

Photo by Lisa Benn

OUR STORY

I am an award winning northern California travel author who has sold over 100,000 books and generated millions of dollars in tourist revenue which trickles from 100's of mom and pop businesses to every corner of the north coast economy.

Because I am a 100% disabled Vietnam Vet I could use the GI Bill to buy a farm in 2016. My home is Be Kind Farm located near the Mendocino Coast. Everyone living on Be Kind Farm was rescued from homelessness. We are all clean and sober doers who have each others back, know what we have and are very grateful. We help some of our friends and neighbors with organic GMO free broccoli, salad greens, heirloom tomatoes and strawberries which we grow in our rich regenerative black soil or in pots in the greenhouse.

The idea for this book came from listening to the radio in 2021. The announcer said that some children in Fort Bragg were going to bed hungry. When I heard that I cried. I decided to do a local guidebook that would strengthen the safety net of food and shelter providers and help local families. Partnering over 100 mom and pop tourist oriented businesses featured in the Mendocino Dining and Lodging Guidebook with a network of non profits benefiting people and animals and 20 local churches with tourist revenue would help. Thats my story.

You can enjoy my travel website at http://www.northofsf.com Please hit the donate button on the home or contact page as this helps Be Kind Farm and with publishing bills. Travel with Love, Gratitude and Kindness and enjoy our beautiful Mendocino Coast. Thank You and Happy Travels !!

The Magic of Westport

Dine here
Enjoy a mocha or smoothie
at Siren's Cafe, high tea,
craft beer, premium wine
or gourmet dinner at the
Westport Hotel and hot coffee,
pizza or sandwich at the Westport Store

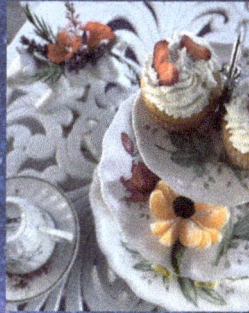

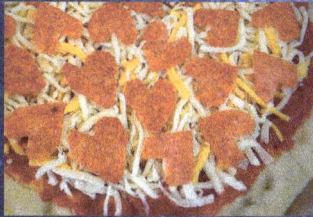

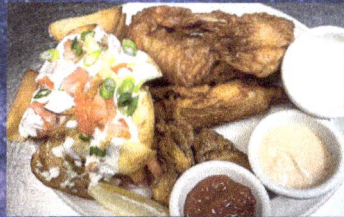

Stay at
Howard Creek Ranch,
the Lost Coast Vista Inn,
Wages Creek Campground
or the elegant Westport Hotel.
Enjoy dramatic Pacific vistas
here on the edge of the Lost Coast. . . .

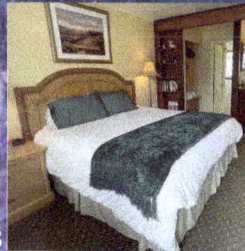

TRAVEL NOTES